Coping with HIV Infection

Psychological and Existential Responses in Gay Men

AIDS Prevention and Mental Health

Series Editors:

David G. Ostrow, M.D., Ph.D.
Howard Brown Health Center and University of Illinois/Chicago School of Public Health, Chicago, Illinois

Jeffrey A. Kelly, Ph.D.
Center for AIDS Intervention Research (CAIR), Milwaukee, Wisconsin

---

Coping with HIV Infection:
Psychological and Existential Responses in Gay Men
Lena Nilsson Schönnesson and Michael W. Ross

Evaluating HIV Prevention Interventions
Joanne E. Mantell, Ph.D., M.S.P.H., Anthony T. DiVittis, M.A., and Marilyn I. Auerbach, A.M.L.S., Dr. P.H.

Handbook of Economic Evaluation of HIV Prevention Programs
Edited by David R. Holtgrave, Ph.D.

Methodological Issues in AIDS Behavioral Research
Edited by David G. Ostrow, M.D., Ph.D., and Ronald C. Kessler. Ph.D.

Preventing AIDS: Theories and Methods of Behavioral Interventions
Edited by Ralph J. DiClemente, Ph.D., and John L. Peterson, Ph.D.

Preventing HIV in Developing Countries:
Biomedical and Behavioral Approaches
Edited by Laura Gibney, Ph.D., Ralph J. DiClemente, Ph.D., and Sten H. Vermund, Ph.D., M.D.

Psychosocial and Public Health Impacts of New HIV Therapies
Edited by David G. Ostrow, M.D., Ph.D., and Seth C. Kalichman, Ph.D.

Social Networks, Drug Injectors' Lives and HIV/AIDS
Samuel R. Friedman, Ph.D., Richard Curtis, Ph.D., Alan Neaigus, Ph.D., Benny Jose, Ph.D., and Don D. Des Jarlais, Ph.D.

Women and AIDS: Coping and Care
Edited by Ann O'Leary, Ph.D., and Lorretta Sweet Jemmott, R.N., Ph.D., F.A.A.N.

Women at Risk: Issues in the Primary Prevention of AIDS
Edited by Ann O'Leary, Ph.D., and Lorretta Sweet Jemmott, R.N., Ph.D.

A Continuation Order Plan is available for this series. A continuation order will bring delivery of each new volume immediately upon publication. Volumes are billed only upon actual shipment. For further information please contact the publisher.

Coping with HIV Infection

Psychological and Existential Responses in Gay Men

Lena Nilsson Schönnesson

Department of Social Work
University of Gothenburg
Gothenburg, Sweden

and

Michael W. Ross

WHO Center for Health Promotion Research and Development
School of Public Health
University of Texas, Houston Health Science Center
Houston, Texas

Springer Science+Business Media, LLC

Library of Congress Cataloging-in-Publication Data

Schönnesson, Lena Nilsson.
Coping with HIV infection : psychological and existential responses in gay men / Lena Nilsson Schönnesson and Michael W. Ross.
p. cm. -- (AIDS prevention and mental health)
Includes bibliographical references and index.
ISBN 978-1-4613-7119-9 ISBN 978-1-4615-4681-8 (eBook)
DOI 10.1007/978-1-4615-4681-8
1. AIDS (Disease)--Psychological aspects. 2. Gay men--Mental health. 3. AIDS (Disease)--Patients--Counseling of. 4. Gay men--Counseling of. 5. Existential psychotherapy. 6. Psychodynamic psychotherapy. I. Ross, Michael W., 1952- . II. Title. III. Series.
RC607.A26S3735 1999
616.97'92'0086642--dc21 99-38194
CIP

ISBN 978-1-4613-7119-9

Originally published by Kluwer Academic / Plenum Publishers in 1999
Softcover reprint of the hardcover 1st edition 1999

All is tender, all is caressed by hands,
God himself blots out the distant lands.
All is near, and all is from afar.
Loaned to man all
Beauteous things that are.

Pär Lagerkvist
From *Beauty Fills Us*
Translation by G. Kenneth Laycock
and Martin S. Allwood, 1950

Foreword

"I'm like a whirling leaf in the wind," said one of Dr. Lena Nilsson Schönnesson's patients, and another "I'm in the claws of HIV." Their voices and those of other HIV-positive patients frame the humanistic and scholarly discussion in this important book. Dr. Schönnesson, a Fulbright scholar at the HIV Center for Clinical and Behavioral Studies, Columbia University in 1995, has unusually extensive clinical experience in counseling HIV-positive gay men. Her work with 38 such patients treated between 1986 and 1995 is discussed in the pages that follow. Dr. Schönnesson's *longitudinal* approach to clinical data is extremely unusual in the psychotherapy literature generally, and in the literature on counseling HIV-positive men in particular. Building upon the experience of such recent scholar-clinicians as Klitzman, Isay, Schaffner, and others, Dr. Schönnesson adds something unique by analyzing her ongoing detailed notes of the psychotherapeutic process in a systematic quantitative as well as qualitative manner. The analysis of her data is further informed by her coauthor, Dr. Michael Ross, a therapist and investigator whose contribution to the clinical and research literature on the psychotherapeutic treatment of gay men has already been substantial.

Dr. Schönnesson's approach to psychotherapy may perhaps be best described as psychodynamic/existential. The conceptual model she relies on to clarify underlying themes are predominately those of self-psychology supplemented by the insights of Winnicott, Sullivan, and modern clinicians experienced in psychotherapeutic work with gay men. Therapists unfamiliar with Kohut's writings will find his important ideas about mirroring, twinship, and idealization explained clearly yet elegantly. Experienced self psychologists and psychoanalysts will find Dr. Schönnesson's application of these constructs to ameliorate the suffering of her patients illuminating.

Respecting complexity at every turn, the authors are able to view behavioral patterns across and within individuals. Ever sensitive to the impact of the physical symptoms of HIV-related diseases, they analyze data in terms of four degrees of severity of illness: asymptomatic, mildly symptomatic, severely symptomatic, and terminal.

Without using jargon they eloquently discuss narratives of 38 individuals who felt "persecuted" by powerful, sometimes overwhelming forces. The tendency for patients' to feel violated often leads to rage at the many treatments they must endure. One comments: "All these pills are poisoned and sooner or later they will kill me." The demands placed not only on the patients but also on the medical and behavioral health professionals who treat them are considerable.

Throughout this volume, Drs. Schönnesson and Ross discuss the similarities and differences between gay men who are HIV positive and patients with non-HIV-related chronic, serious diseases, especially cancer. A major difference concerns issues specific to being gay. Virtually all the men in this sample had to confront and overcome stigmatization and prejudice because of their homosexual orientation. For many, becoming HIV positive led to resurgence of conflicts about being gay that had previously been put to rest. The patients were faced with often painful decisions about disclosure of their HIV status—a second "coming out" process. Sometimes the responses of those in their social surround were disappointing and the circle of supportive others diminished. The ensuing feelings of disillusionment and anger were expressed and coped with in psychotherapy.

The patients discussed in this volume were treated prior to the very recent surge of progress in pharmacotherapy of HIV. Foreshortened life expectancy and coping with impending death are major themes of this book. Even therapists who are experienced in working with terminal patients will learn much from the authors' clinical wisdom. Discussion of the treatment of Steven, a patient treated with psychotherapy for six years until his death, poignantly illustrates this. At the end of his life Dr. Schönnesson sometimes fed Steven, listened to music with him, read to him, and at times the two simply sat together in silence. The reader feels privileged to learn about dignified people involved in an empathic, professional relationship discussed in simple straightforward prose.

One might wonder whether a volume devoted to such weighty matters might not be depressing to read. To the contrary, this book is inspiring because it is primarily about the challenges and rewards of living well in the face of adversity. In the words of the authors, "the quality of life is the ultimate goal of the adaptation process." Sexuality is a theme especially emphasized; its many meanings to gay men, the difficulties of accepting limitations on sexual expressiveness because of being HIV positive, the necessity to cope with loss of sexual functions, the rewards and pleasure of sexual love, the difficulties in relationships when one partner is HIV positive and the other is not.

Freud recognized that intimate relationships are inherently ambivalent, an insight that has been validated by future generations of psychotherapists. This is certainly true of psychotherapeutic relationships, and especially so for the unique relationships between HIV-positive patients and their therapists. One of Dr. Schönnesson's patient's described her as being "an unpleasant pleasure."

An important psychotherapeutic principle affirmed in this volume is that a caring, present psychotherapist can help a patient stabilize his self-representation and improve the quality of life under trying and even desperate circumstances. All clinicians and psychotherapy researchers will learn something from this book, but especially those working with gay men.

RICHARD C. FRIEDMAN, M.D.
Clinical Professor of Psychiatry, Cornell University Medical College
New York City, NY

Preface

The impetus and the source of inspiration of writing this book is my (Dr. Schönnesson's) psychotherapeutic work in Stockholm, Sweden, with gay men living with HIV since 1986. The men have shared with me their worries and concerns as well as the enigmatic existential issues related to HIV disease. Many of them had reached the peak of imbalance between the HIV-related burdens and their available resources, experiencing hopelessness, negative resignation, existing but not living, and being stuck in the HIV trauma and its mourning. They expressed a wish to change the HIV scenario from one of a desert to a flourishing oasis, in which they celebrate themselves and their lives. Another desire has been to assign HIV "the right proportion" in their lives. As one man said, "You know, I don't want all my books in my bookshelves to be on HIV." In the course of our psychotherapeutic work, the gay men have also become curious about exploring further their internal landscapes and their authentic selves.

The prime motive for writing this book has been the wish to share my clinical experiences and to let the men's voices be heard. It is of great significance to listen to the gay men's own words in describing and illuminating the spectrum and complexity of the HIV scenario and all of its adaptational tasks and challenges and their impact on the individual's self. In contrast to empirical HIV-related psychosocial research, which mostly is cross-sectional, the long-term longitudinal character of the clinical data presented in this book makes it possible to examine long-term HIV adaptation. Another void that this book will start to fill, we hope, is the minimal understanding of inner psychological experiences and processes of gay men with HIV and their changes over the disease phases. The book parts from most other HIV-related research in that HIV disease is considered within the context of the individual's self and the existential frame of reference. We firmly believe that these two contexts are of vital importance in order to deepen and broaden our understanding of what it means to be gay and to live with HIV disease.

It is our hope that what is to be read in the following pages will serve as an inspiration to therapists and counselors to acclaim the role that they can play in supporting the individual to achieve psychological integration and hope in the face of HIV disease.

Acknowledgments

In writing any book, there is always one debt that stands out above all the others. In our case, that debt is to the men who are the source of the stories contained here. Indeed, without them, this book would not have been written, and we thank them for what they have taught us.

Nor would this book have been as complete without the detailed assistance of three collaborators. Dr. Kerstin Fugl-Meyer, of the Department of Sexology, University Hospital, Uppsala, Sweden, cowrote Chapter 9 and provided enormous support in corating all the psychotherapeutic sessions as well as the case histories for the qualitative analysis and discussing them in detail over a considerable period of time. Dr. Curtis Dolezal, of the HIV Center for Clinical and Behavioral Studies at Columbia University, New York, carried out the organization of the data by disease phases and the quantitative analyses reported here. He responded with great patience and support to numerous calls and faxes requesting additional analyses and clarification. Eva Edvardson, at the PH-Center in Stockholm, spent hours entering the coded session sheets into the Statistical Package for the Social Sciences (SPSS) file.

No book is possible without strong and consistent support from employers and colleagues. This book was made possible by a research grant (1996 7187) from the Department of Research, Education and Development at Stockholm City Council to Dr. Lena Nilsson Schönnesson, and by a leave of absence from the PH-Center in Stockholm. It was also supported by a study leave to Dr. Michael Ross from the University of Texas—School of Public Health, to work at Gothenburg University, Sweden. Finally, to all those who contributed in so many ways, named and unnamed, go our thanks and gratitude.

Contents

1

Living on the Boundaries

Retrospectively, various diseases such as leprosy, the plague, and tuberculosis have evoked fear, disgust, repudiation, but also stigmatization of the afflicted person. Their equivalent of today is HIV infection. As we write this, the HIV epidemic has raged for over 20 years and has been known about for 17 years. The natural disease process is relatively well understood and the secrets of the virus are being unlocked by science. Yet, an equivalent understanding of the psychological, social, and sexual aspects of the drama of HIV infection and its psychological landscapes in which it is embedded has been slower in coming. Unlike the response of the body to HIV infection, which has a more finite range of possibilities, the response of the person with HIV to their condition may encompass a wide range of reactions and adaptations across their life span and across the phases of the disease.

The focus of this book is to describe and illuminate the drama of HIV in view of the disease process among gay men and the psychological landscapes in which it is embedded. It concentrates on gay men not only because of HIV's first appearance in the United States, Scandinavia, and Western Europe in this community, but also because those who have been longest infected are in this group. The gay experience brings with it a unique set of psychological issues, which HIV disease may echo, and for this reason, we do not deal with women or nongay men with HIV disease. Although this book has an individualistic approach, we firmly believe that it is critical to view gay men living with HIV within a societal context of antigay attitudes and stigmatization. Without such awareness the empathy and understanding of the gay man with HIV is limited.

The psychological landscapes of gay men with HIV are indeed familiar to us, in that we have both had the opportunity of working as psychotherapists (and researchers) with gay men with HIV disease since the early 1980s. I (Dr. Schönnesson) have been working with gay men with HIV disease in Stockholm—in many cases seeing men from the time of first awareness of their infection until their death or in their continuing life with HIV. For both of us, our research and clinical work was primarily with gay men before the emergence of HIV.

STRUCTURE OF THE BOOK

The book is divided into two broader sections. Chapters 2 through 6 focus on the HIV scenario. They include the notification of HIV diagnosis, physical, social, and sexual threats, and their concomitant psychological issues as well as their impact on psychological functioning and quality of life. In Chapters 7 through 9, the psychological landscapes of the HIV scenario are addressed. From our perspective, the concept of psychological landscape serves as a frame of reference to better understand and appreciate the meaning of living with HIV. The individual psychological landscape corresponds to the existential, the adaptation, and the self contexts. As these contexts may vary among individuals and over the disease phases, it appears to be more appropriate to talk about landscape in plurals rather than in singular. The final chapter of the book ties together some of the major themes that arise in the preceding two sections.

The illustration of the HIV scenario and the psychological landscapes is comprised of a combination of empirical and quantitatively and qualitatively clinical data (see "Methodology" in this chapter). The latter is based on Dr. Schönnesson's longitudinal psychotherapeutic notes of gay men with HIV. However, there are two exceptions to the combination principle; Chapter 2, "The Impact of Chronic and Terminal Illness," which is a strictly theoretical chapter, and Chapter 3, "HIV Testing and Its Impact," in which only empirical data are presented. As the purpose of the book is to describe and analyze the HIV scenario and its psychological landscapes across the phases of the disease, the clinical material was organized accordingly. A short summary of each chapter is provided below.

Chapter 2, "The Impact of Chronic and Terminal Illness," incorporates HIV disease into a broader illness perspective. It is a purely theoretical chapter in which a host of disease and adaptation models are presented to highlight common elements of people with HIV disease with those with other chronic or terminal diseases such as cancer, which is alluded to throughout the book. But there are also the unique elements, which are brought to HIV not only by its newness and epidemiology, but also by the previous experiences of stigmatization in gay men.

Chapter 3, "HIV Testing and Its Impact." The HIV scenario and its drama begin at the moment the individual decides to test for HIV and discovers he is HIV seropositive and it ends only with death. HIV testing, notification of HIV seroconversion, and psychological reactions are described in the chapter. We also discuss the effect of testing on sexual behaviors and self-disclosure of serostatus.

Chapter 4, "HIV-Related Threats." The drama of the HIV scenario circles around its ongoing potential threats toward the individual's physical, social, and sexual existences. The virus not only threatens the person's physical but also psychological survival. His social existence is threatened in terms of potential discrimination and aloneness (i.e., social death), which are the negative consequences of disclosing one's HIV status. But his social existence is also threatened by loss of friends to HIV disease. Finally, the person's sexual existence is exposed to HIV-related physical/medical, social, and psychological threats (i.e., sexual death).

In Chapter 5, "The Insidious Persecutory Drama of HIV," various psychological issues, which are undoubtedly a response to the variety of HIV-related threats, are discussed. These issues are persecution, death anxiety, existential death anxiety and death awareness, loss and mourning, control, despair versus hope, and psychological defenses.

Chapter 6, "The Impact of HIV Infection on Psychological Functioning and Quality of Life." People with HIV respond to HIV-related threats and psychological issues in a broad range of modes partly as a result of their adaptation processes. The mode spectrum varies from psychiatric disorders to transient mood symptoms. The reactions may vary over time and be dependent on the character of the threat. We also focus on the impact of HIV infection on quality of life and the influence of psychological and social stress mediators.

In Chapters 7 through 9 the focus is on the psychological landscapes in which HIV disease is embedded.

Chapter 7, "The Existential Context." We suggest that a vital prerequisite for understanding the meaning of the HIV drama is its existential context within a philosophical frame of reference in terms of death, freedom, isolation, and meaning. In this chapter each of these existential concerns are discussed and illuminated.

In Chapter 8, "HIV Adaptation Processes," we focus on the second component of the psychological landscape, that is, the adaptation processes of HIV-related threats and psychological issues. We discuss briefly the approaches of psychosocial variables and stage models in describing the individual's HIV adaptation process. We believe, however, that a spiral approach, based on the concept of psychological metabolism, does more justice to the complexity of the adaptation process. The approach is described and illuminated.

Chapter 9, "The Shattered Self," is centered on the individual's self, encompassing self-image and self-esteem. The self, which is the third part of the individual's psychological landscape, can be viewed as a filter through which HIV-related threats and psychological issues are mediated and understood. However, various psychological stressors compromise the self and, as the title of the chapter infers, the consequence is a more or less shattered self. Just as the gay men struggle with adapting to the HIV-related threats and psychological issues, they also struggle with processing and restoring their more or less shattered self. As is described in the chapter, the men use different approaches in their attempt to restore it. One approach is through their social network and another is through psychotherapeutic relationship. We suggest that the HIV-disease adaptation processes interplay with the self-adaptation processes and that they are both embedded in the existential context of death, freedom, isolation, and meaning.

In the final chapter, "Autonomy, Boundaries, Control, and Death," we summarize the most salient aspects of the insidious persecutory drama of the HIV scenario and its psychological landscapes over the disease phases. We also address clinical implications of our findings as well as psychotherapeutic issues.

METHODOLOGY

In order to describe and illuminate the HIV scenario and its psychological landscapes we have used three methodological approaches—review of previous empirical work and quantitative and qualitative methods in analyzing Dr. Schönnesson's longitudinal psychotherapeutic notes of 38 gay men, from a sample of 88, with HIV. The methodology of the study is presented in the Appendix. This methodological approach is founded upon the need to provide as many perspectives from which to allow triangulation and an assessment of the reliability and similarity of the experiences of these men. We hope that using all three methodological approaches will provide a degree of rigor, which may have been lacking with the use of only one of these.

With respect to empirical work from other researchers in the area, we combine in a relatively seamless way reports from the United States, Europe, and Australia. In the quantitative analysis of the psychotherapeutic notes, we identify frequency and intensity of the themes that emerged in the course of psychotherapy with these men and also the different phases of the disease process at which they emerged and retreated.

The notes were further qualitatively analyzed within an existential, self psychology, and object-relations and disease-phases perspective. A staging classification, which was scored by Dr. Schönnesson on the basis on the individual's description of his health status, was used to represent the disease phases. Phase 1 refers to the asymptomatic phase (an "intact" immune system, no symptoms) and phase 2 to the mild symptomatic phase (a somewhat impaired immune system with mild symptoms). Phase 3 refers to the severe symptomatic phase (impaired immune system and severe symptoms) and phase 4 to the terminal phase. Those quotes and examples of gay men that are provided in the book are, unless otherwise stated, drawn from psychotherapeutic notes. We also want to underscore that the words that are shared by the gay men with HIV are authentic in that they are not psychodynamically interpreted. The names that are being used in quotes, examples, case studies, and case vignettes have been chosen randomly and there is no personal connection between the various quotes with the exception of the three cases in Chapter 8 and 9. We chose this approach to protect the gay men's anonymity and confidentiality. That we approach the issue of the psychological issues involved in living with HIV primarily from the psychodynamic perspective does not of course exclude the importance or significance of looking at psychological issues of living with HIV for gay men through other lenses.

We recognize that criticism could be raised in that these men attended psychotherapeutic counseling, and thus they may have been atypical in their need to work through their issues in living and dying with HIV. They may also be reflecting the processes of working through issues in a therapeutic setting in their progress in dealing with the disease. We have no comparison group to answer this question and doubt if one would be ethically acceptable even if available. Nevertheless, the men who tell us their stories in these pages bring up the same themes we have heard in our clinical and research work from gay men living with HIV in Sweden, the United States, and Australia. The psychological issues that arise in these geographically diverse but essentially modern Judeo-Christian first world cultures are quite similar. However, we are aware of the fact that the United States almost alone among Western civilizations has no comprehensive universal health care system, which does impose an additional burden on many gay men who have no or inadequate insurance or who are unemployed. The fact that the right to adequate health care and treatment is denied to many in the United States will add a layer of uncertainty and distress to the process of HIV disease in many gay men in the United States that we cannot capture here. Another aspect that is more salient among urban gay men in the United States is their heavy confrontation with multiple losses of friends to HIV and bereavement, which adds another stressor of major concern.

TIME AND BOUNDARIES

Time is at the core of this work. Various aspects of time—time as people proceed from asymptomatic disease through mild and later severe symptoms to the terminal phase of the disease. Time as people adapt to their condition and deal with the issues, which have been thrust into consciousness by the infection. Time as the scientific and medical world better understand and control the disease process, from AZT (azidothymidine) in the late 1980s to the present regimens of combination therapies with protease inhibitors. Time as people with HIV get older and deal with HIV as it interacts with the issues raised by aging and career progression. Time as people deal with the reactions of others, such as lovers, friends, and family, which will themselves also alter with the progress of time.

The second issue, which has arisen in the course of this work, is the issue of boundaries as central to the process of dealing with HIV disease. The centrality of this theme emerged subtly as this book took shape, culminating in the realization that the uncertainty of the disease process and many of the questions that the people we worked with related to boundaries. The boundaries included not only the nebulous boundaries between chronic and terminal disease, between illness and health, and between hope and despair, but the ultimate boundary of death and the existential concerns that all of these raised. One of the stressors of living with HIV is the lack of precision of these boundaries and the uncertainty as to which side one may be on—as well as the need to set boundaries in many aspects of life and relationships. For this reason, we used as the title of this chapter Barnard's[1] expression of the experience of "living on the boundaries." Because of its centrality it could also be another subtitle of this work.

Objections might be raised that the voices of the gay men in this book are illustrative of another era of the HIV history, as the vast majority of the psychotherapeutic material was "collected" prior to protease inhibitors and combination therapies. But we would argue that many of the issues that these men (as well as those who participated in all the empirical studies) faced are the same as those who are diagnosed with HIV today. We strongly question whether the stigma of HIV has significantly changed, but surely the sexual dilemmas still exist. The uncertainty is still there although it has changed its gestalt. In the early days of HIV, the uncertainty was about "when will I die," including death anxiety. Today uncertainty is about "how long will I live," which to some induces life anxiety. At the bottom line, the new medications are no guarantee of certainty. The only certainty that does exist is that we will all die, regardless of HIV status. So the individual continues to face existential issues, including death anxiety. The need to adapt to HIV-related threats and various psychological issues, to restore a more or less shattered self, and to experience quality of life is an ongoing process and that will not change because of protease inhibitors. To quote Klitzman: "New drugs help, but they aren't enough."[2]

At the end of all this, however, we believe that this book is about the intensely personal experiences of the men who we have been privileged to work with over the past 15 years. We have tried to personalize what is after all an intensely personal process—the way people deal with the uncertainties of living on physical, psychological, and temporal boundaries. We believe that what will breathe life into this work is the authentic voices of the men who have lived and died or still live with HIV disease, and we are grateful to them for sharing their lives with us.

REFERENCES

1. Barnard D. Chronic illness and the dynamics of hoping. In: Toombs SK, Barnard D, Carson RA, eds. *Chronic Illness: From Experience to Policy.* Bloomington: Indiana University Press, 1995; 38–57.
2. Klitzman R. *Being Positive: The Lives of Men and Women with HIV.* Chicago: Ivan R. Dee; 1997.

I

The HIV Scenario

2

The Impact of Chronic and Terminal Illness

HIV disease does not occur in a vacuum from other illness processes, both chronic and terminal. As a consequence, a significant amount of what we know about responses to, and impact of, chronic and terminal illnesses has relevance to HIV disease. On the other hand, the pandemic in predominantly gay men in the 1980s in North America and Western Europe also brought a number of unique features into the situation, among them the collective experience of the gay subculture, the stigmatization resulting from the co-categorization of male gayness and AIDS, and the experience of dealing with the stigmatization of a gay orientation. This chapter explores both the common and unique elements of dealing with HIV disease in this population.

One of the initially unique aspects of HIV in the first few years of the pandemic was its newness—a new disease, a newly discovered virus, and the lack of knowledge of the natural history of the disease process. There was no "illness narrative" that provided a model as to how to deal with the disease or indeed of its progression, and certainly no model of a pandemic that attacked a specific class of persons who were in the prime of their lives and often well educated and politically organized. Thus, the construction of the meaning of the disease in the Western world was a joint production between the medical profession and the affected community. The magnitude of what was unknown set the stage for the development of a mythology and an iconography of majestic dimensions, as well as provided a remarkable latitude for both hope and despair.

Further, as Barnard[1] argues, chronic illness is an attack on the self. Humans have a symbolic identity, and chronic illness has an impact on that identity. Where symbolic identity is constructed upon a self-concept and a history, the impact of a major illness, which is chronic or terminal and disabling of that identity constitutes an existential challenge. And, we believe, a disease process that is tied so closely to an identity is by its very nature likely to, as Barnard argues, "call attention to a dialectic within human beings' self awareness." He refers to this as "the experience of living on the boundary"[1] (p. 39)—the boundary of a unique identity, and the frailty and ultimate mortality of that identity, between transcendence and finitude.

This existential paradox of chronic illness, Barnard suggests, is integral to the dynamics of hoping and despair. There can be a demoralizing confrontation with unavoidable limitations and loss occasioned by chronic illness—and the "re-moralization"[2] and kindling of hope. Barnard notes that "the tension between remoralization and demoralization is another way of expressing the intimate connection between hope and despair; it is the emotional counterpart to the more abstract, metaphysical concept of reconciling possibility and necessity"[1] (p. 40). These existential tensions are at the heart of any response to chronic and terminal illness. We do not see "chronic" and "terminal" illness as necessarily exclusive terms. An illness may be chronic but not terminal, terminal but not chronic, neither, or both. Chronicity refers to its not being time-limited, but as being expected to continue, while terminal suggests a worsening toward an inevitable death in the foreseeable future. This difference is essentially one in speed and trajectory. It could be summed up as a difference between "living with the disease" and "dying of the disease."

The chronically ill person, according to Murphy[3] emphasizes the liminality, or boundary phenomenon, of illness—the chronically ill are human but their bodies are warped or malfunctioning, leaving their full humanity in doubt—and illness is transitional to either death or recovery. He suggests that the sick person lives in a state of social suspension until he or she gets better (or dies). Such a condition of suspended humanity or incomplete humanity may serve to alienate (or further alienate) the ill from their social spheres. Thus, uncertainty, alienation, despair, and hope may form a background for response to illness.

In her work with breast cancer, Taylor[4] reports three recurring themes associated with coping with the news of the diagnosis: a search for meaning, an attempt to regain control over their lives, and an effort to enhance self-esteem. Barnard argues that each of these goals involves some modifications in the woman's perceptions of reality, in that "illusions"—of certainty of causation, of control over illness progression, of self-enhancing social comparisons—become the material of coping. He argues that those who cope best with their cancer were sustained by unrealistically positive views of their personal control of themselves, and the order and meaning in events (that is, by illusions). However, in the case of HIV disease, where the predominant meaning of the disease has been expressed in the allusion to punishment, where its occurrence in an already stigmatized and alienated subculture makes it much more difficult to make self-enhancing social comparisons, these factors may actually mitigate against constructive coping.

Nevertheless, Barnard suggests that an understanding of the dynamics of hoping may rest on the concept of illusion, which rests between the domains of "hard facts" and hallucination. He describes this as the "realm of play, culture, and imagination. In this sphere there is the constant interplay between internal images and external objects, between personal gropings toward meaning and the affirmations and corrections of culturally available formulations"[1] (p. 49). The realm of illusion is precisely that realm explored by psychotherapy, where the illumination of the shifting meaning across the process of the disease as well as through the processes of adaptation situates our attempts to understand living with HIV disease.

Psychotherapy is also the illumination of the stories of living (and dying) with HIV disease. Barnard argues that the illness experience is a story, and that the dynamics of hoping and despair that will underlie coping and adaptation amount to what may be called the "renarratization" of illness[1] (p. 53). We argue that throughout the temporal course of all of these processes—the disease process, the treatment process, and the adaptation process—coping and adaptation can be understood by the changing narratives and by the foci of these narratives. Adaptation and coping are dynamic processes in interplay that are illuminated by these narratives and "renarratives." We discuss the concepts of coping and adaptation in more detail in Chapters 6 and 8, respectively. Such narratives need to be seen in a broader context, as Brody states, that of the "life plan."[5] Brody analyzes several classic works of literature dealing with illness and finds that there is a list of possible "stories of sickness." First, sickness may be viewed as a gap in one's life plans, and when it is over, one takes up these plans where one left off. Second, one can pursue one's life plan as if nothing has happened—until the illness becomes too severe to be ignored. Third, Brody suggests, is the story of adopting sickness as one's career, abandoning one's previous life plan and formulating a new one with sickness as a centerpiece. Fourth, if the illness is seen as progressive or fatal, one may pursue one's life plan without major modification, only accelerating its pace given the short time remaining. Fifth, sickness may force a modification of one's life plan, so that the time after the sickness is diagnosed is followed by a reexamination and a formulation of a new life plan that is rational given the limitations that the chronic sickness is expected to impose. Sixth, Brody argues, it is possible that the old life plan was such a major part of one's self that to lose it is to lose one's identity—after the illness diagnosis, the story is of an entirely different individual. Finally, sickness can be seen as a jarring note, which makes a mockery of the life plan that has gone before, or as the natural close of a long and fruitful life.

These scenarios, however, presuppose that there is a "life plan" that illness is superimposed upon. Where there is no life plan to define one's existence, other existential crises may yet emerge. For example, if one's existence is based upon a sexual-orientation identity (e.g., self-definition as gay) and one's value is based in terms of sexual capital, then there may be a "life meaning" rather than a "life plan." Such a "life meaning" may, however, also lead to similar continuations, interruptions, and redefinitions. The meaning of the life as lived to the point of diagnosis, and the meaning of the illness, may produce a dialectic in which the synthesis is the adjustment to the disease. This is particularly likely to be the case, we argue, where both the lifestyle and the disease are pregnant with meaning.

Sontag[6] describes the meaning of an illness as the punitive or sentimental fantasies concocted about the situation of that illness—and uses tuberculosis (TB) and cancer, and to a lesser extent syphilis, as examples of diseases with significantly different meanings attached. She argues that such chronic (and until recently terminal) disease has been regarded as a synonym for death: "The metaphors attached to TB and to cancer imply living processes of a particularly resonant and horrid kind"[6] (p. 9). Cancer implies an invasion and a death of fear and agony, while syphilis, because of the clearer understanding of its causation, transmission, and treatment, contains an implicit moral, rather than psychological, judgment. In the case of cancer and TB, she argues, there is an implied psychological judgment contained: in the case of cancer, associated with repression; in the case of TB, with creativity.

One of the more pervasive notions associated with illness, Sontag[6] argues, is seeing disease as an instrument of divine wrath, either at a community level for epidemics, or at an individual level. If there is a preconception of disease as punishment for wickedness, then it is more likely that the meaning of the illness will stress moral corruption. In such cases, the disease will be seen as an appropriate and just punishment, she suggests, quoting Groddeck: "The sick man himself creates his disease. He is the cause of the disease and we need seek no other" (p. 46). However, the meanings attached to diseases may allow no escape from the belief that the cause of illness is located in the individual: if one has cancer, it is because one has loved too little or repressed love; if syphilis, one has loved too much. Meaning is almost impossible to avoid and, as Sontag notes, has a stigmatizing effect at the public level and a condemnatory impact at the personal level: "Nothing is more punitive than to give disease a meaning—that meaning being invariably a moralistic one"[6] (p. 58). Disease itself then becomes a metaphor.

Further, Sontag[7] argues, illnesses have traditionally been used as metaphors to enliven charges that a society was corrupt or unjust. In the case of HIV disease/AIDS, she suggests, the meaning extends: to have AIDS in one of the countries where homosexual transmission (or injecting drug use) accounts for the majority of cases is to be revealed as a member of a community of pariahs, and flushes out an identity that might have remained hidden. She extends the traditional meanings associated with disease, in the case of AIDS, to a greater degree of blame—its being more willfully acquired, and thus associated with greater guilt, as well as afflicting the already-stigmatized.

These meanings, it must be emphasized, are imposed and bear no relationship to medical reality: TB, HIV, and syphilis, to use a few examples, are contracted through infection with a virulent pathogen. Nor does cancer have any implications for personality: it results from damaging mutations in the replication mechanisms of body cells, in some cases initiated or promoted through contact with toxic substances. The arbitrariness of the imposition of a punitive and moralistic meaning on a disease process is highlighted by Butler's *Erewhon*,[8] a satirical novel. It describes a society in which criminal activity is seen as being equivalent to sickness and treated sympathetically with bed rest, and in which illness is seen as equivalent to crime and punished with a severity related to the severity of the illness, including imprisonment.

Illness concepts (or meanings) will be intimately associated with the patient's response to the illness and their long-term coping strategies. Lipowski[9] described eight different illness concepts in patients based on clinical experience: (1) illness as a challenge (insightful acceptance); (2) illness as an enemy; (3) illness as punishment; (4) illness as weakness; (5) illness as relief; (6) illness as strategy; (7) illness as irreparable loss or damage; and (8) illness as value. He argued that the significance of a chronic illness to the patient reflects this personal meaning (which may be conscious, but not necessarily so). We use the term "meaning" here as referring to a dynamic process. It may commence with the translation of the disease into concepts already used and understood by the individual; that is, the construction of a psychological explanatory system around the disease in order to make sense of it. "Meaning" also connotes the subjective representation of or the symbolic attribution to HIV and even its adoption as an identity.

Empirical support for Lipowski's meanings of illness was provided by Schüssler,[10] who looked at over 200 patients with chronic illnesses, and reported that many of Lipowski's eight illness concepts were interrelated. He also looked at controllability and coping styles, and found that the more an illness endangers self-esteem, the more threatening it is. Illness as challenge (insightful acceptance), illness as value, and a sense of internal control were connected with more favorable coping factors, such as cognitive reconstruction and giving meaning to the illness. Concepts of illness as enemy, illness as punishment, and illness as relief are associated with negative emotional coping, wishful thinking, and psychologically immature defenses. Illness as strategy leads to active coping strategies. Two different types of social modes of illness-meaning related coping were found: negative coping, including social withdrawal; and cognitive reconstruction, connected with emotional stability, self-efficacy, and social competence.

Schüssler also found that there were psychological consequences associated with illness meanings, with seeing illness as enemy or illness as punishment associated with depression and anxiety. Interestingly, he concluded that there is no disease concept that is specific to a chronic illness, and that in order to favorably deal with a disease, moderate denial (specifically, their threat potential and their uncertainty) is necessary. Further, the level of perceived controllability is important: if the sick person has the feeling of being able to influence their illness, then more active and problem-associated coping strategies are used. Thus, emotion-based coping is more likely to occur in people who do not accept their illness or do not consider it to be controllable. These data demonstrate clearly that illness concepts and meanings have a decisive influence on coping.

An additional factor associated with response to chronic illness is the illness monitoring process. Miller et al.[11] compared women with precancerous cervical dysplasia to men with HIV disease, dividing their samples into high health monitors (who are cognitively vigilant and amplify threat-related cues) and low monitors (who avoid and blunt their impact). They found that high monitors were characterized by elevated levels of intrusive ideation. They were more likely to think about their disease status when they did not mean to, to dream about it, to have trouble falling asleep because of it, to be reminded of it, and to have strong feelings about it. As a result, they were more likely to engage in avoidance strategies, such as trying not to talk or think about it and staying away from reminders about it, in an attempt to reduce this rumination. As might be expected, high and low monitors had differing strategies for coping with their disease. High monitors are more likely to use denial or disengagement strategies by expending more effort to suppress and distance themselves from an awareness of their situation. While this may be adaptive, allowing the patient to avoid an uncontrollable stressor and reduce stress to a manageable level, denial of the distress and the reality of the situation may mean that they are not able to readily accommodate the reality. Miller et al. note the similarity of this denial and numbing of emotion to post-traumatic stress disorder.

However, the response to HIV infection is a dynamic one: indeed, description of the changes over time in response to HIV disease is the central theme of this book. Asymptomatic people who have tested seropositive for HIV go through a series of adaptation processes and stages of coping with the disease (although as with all stage models, not all stages need be followed consecutively, and some may be missed). Ross, Tebble, and Viliunas[12] based a model of response to HIV infection on clinical observations and interviews with gay men with HIV. Their observations suggested that the stages that were apparent were a combination of Kübler-Ross's[13] stages of death and dying and Cass's[14] model of homosexual identity formation. They noted that the first stage was shock, denial, and anger and feelings of guilt and powerlessness. This was followed by withdrawal: a recognition of the stigma of HIV infection and social isolation. The "bargaining" stage was divided into four substages. These included "coming out" to significant others (testing the reaction of others and recognition of the need to be loved); looking for other HIV-seropositive persons (with a need for sharing, recognition, and social support); turning their alienation into a unique advantage (seeing their status as special and being needed by others); and altruistic behavior (a feeling of community with other HIV-seropositive people). It will be noted that these four substages echo the "coming out" process of gay men, according to Cass. What appears to happen is that gay men may use the lessons and processes learned in coming to terms with one stigmatized status (being gay) to deal with a related stigmatized status (being HIV infected). It follows that the way that such people dealt with their "coming out" is likely to be a model for their coming to terms with their HIV disease, including disclosure to significant others and their wider social environment. Finally, Ross, Tebble, and Viliunas[12] note that a final stage of acceptance in which HIV serostatus is integrated (coming to terms with one's condition) can occur. However, they also note that becoming symptomatic will raise a new set of issues, and that this model is derived solely from asymptomatic men. This model was derived from the responses of gay men in the first five years of the epidemic, and the developments in treatment and the increasing visibility of people with HIV may make the passage through these stages occur more rapidly.

The response of the person with HIV will, however, encompass much more than coming to terms with the infection, which is essentially an internal set of processes. The experience of gay men with HIV disease will reflect their social and cultural context as much as their models of illness and the meanings they attach to their illness. Ross and Ryan,[15] in an extensive qualitative study of perceptions of HIV, sexuality, and quality of life, found that quality of life was dependent on culture and identification, specifically the gay subculture and identification of the infection with their gay identity and behavior. Sex, previously associated with enjoyment and celebration, becomes associated with risk to others and self and responsibility, as well as to a further set of discriminations from their own community. The result may be self-quarantine or the perception or anticipation of sexual rejection. The attribution of their sexuality as being responsible for becoming infected with HIV may lead to feeling discredited and self-doubtful (a modified version of the meaning of illness as punishment or guilt-associated).

Quality of life issues in HIV-infected gay men, note Ross and Ryan, will include things that are central to the person's definition of self and self-identity, such as, sex and sexuality and sexual relationships. They note that there are two major concepts in gay men that revolve around what they refer to as "the little deaths"—sexual death and social death, which may precede by a considerable time a physical death. Where sexuality is a core identification of homosexually active men, and where sex plays a significant part in maintaining identity and self-esteem, then meaning in life will also involve sexuality. Thus, diminution in sex will involve diminution in quality of life and change in the emphasis of, enjoyment of, or opportunity for expression of sexuality will affect self-definition. However, Ross and Ryan also note a change in emphasis on sexuality for the better—where HIV infection provided a chance to reevaluate one's approach to sexual matters. The physical changes resulting from HIV infection as well as the psychological ones associated with infection may also reduce self-perception of attractiveness and self-confidence, thus leading to social withdrawal.

Ross and Ryan comment that the homosexual is also the homosocial. Much of gay interaction (and thus social support) takes place in gay venues such as bars and clubs. Where there is an emphasis on looks, then there is likely to be rejection, perceived or real, and the person's value (sexual capital) decreases. There may be an anticipatory withdrawal from one's "family of choice" (gay friends), which leads to a degree of "social death." While this will obviously impact social supports and psychological functioning, it also constitutes one area where HIV disease in gay men is significantly different from many other chronic diseases, although as Kübler-Ross has noted for terminal illnesses, there is also a withdrawal stage closer to death. In gay men with HIV disease, Ross and Ryan have cogently argued, this may come much earlier and constitute sexual death and social death, the deaths of two of the most significant social supports—gay identity and self-esteem—in this population. By gay identity we refer simply to the individual's self-identification that they are gay. These themes—sexual death, social death, and physical death—will reemerge in the course of this book.

The stigma associated with HIV disease is unfortunately still one of its defining features, one that sets it aside from almost all other diseases in its degree, although not necessarily by its presence. Some of Ross and Ryan's respondents noted that this "double stigma," being HIV infected and thus stigmatized in the gay community, adds to the social and sexual deaths. Paradoxically, as Ross, Tebble, and Viliunas have also noted, having had the experience of coping with one stigmatized identity (being gay) may provide a useful model for dealing with this second stigmatized identity.

With the progression of disease, attitudes may change. Greer, Morris, and Pettingale[16] found that there were five dimensions of approaching cancer: fighting spirit, anxious preoccupation, helplessness/hopelessness, fatalism, and avoidance. Ross et al.[17] used a modified version of Watson, Greer, and Bliss's Mental Adjustment of Cancer scale[18] to look at response to HIV disease in gay men. Ross et al. found that there were five clearly identifiable dimensions of approaching HIV disease: the first dimension was helplessness/hopelessness, where people felt at a loss as to what to do and out of control of the disease process. The second dimension was fighting spirit, where people had a positive attitude and tried to fight the disease and not let it affect their lives. The third dimension was a belief in being able to influence the course of the disease, like exercise and diet and a positive state of mind. Fourth was denial/avoidance, where people try to avoid finding out too much and take things one day at a time without planning ahead. Finally, there was fatalism/preoccupation, in which people leave it up to others, such as health care workers, and adopt a fatalistic attitude, or alternatively try to gather as much information as possible. What appeared different in the patients with HIV compared with those with cancer was the belief in influencing the course of the disease through exercise, diet, and other modalities—and this dimension was significantly related to fighting spirit.

Helplessness/hopelessness was significantly related to denial/avoidance and fatalism/preoccupation. It thus appears that there are two possible approaches; a positive one of fighting spirit and belief that one could influence the course of the disease; and a negative one, characterized by denial, fatalism, and avoidance. Ross et al.'s data were obtained at the time that AZT was being used to treat HIV disease, but before the advent of protease inhibitors.

The advent of protease inhibitors has lead to an interesting set of responses from those people who had survived HIV disease long enough to benefit from a new class of medications and those who were more recently infected. This parallels the now-famous cases of the "awakenings" first described by Sacks[19] in the early 1970s of people who had been unresponsive and immovable for many decades (resulting from the *Encephalitis lethargica* epidemic following World War I) by the new medication L-DOPA. Sacks has emphasized that the critical aspect of these awakenings was the human side—"what confronted one, ... was not just disease or physiology, but *people*, people struggling to adapt and survive." The central issue was what it was like to "*stay* human, in the face of unimaginable adversities and threats"[19] (p. xxviii). He comments that some of these patients had achieved a state of icy hopelessness akin to serenity (a realistic hopelessness); some had a fierce and impotent sense of outrage for being swindled out of the best years of life and consumed by a sense of time lost or wasted. They wanted to be given back the lost time and to be magically replaced in their youth and prime. Sacks argues that what is lost, in a metaphysical sense, in those who are sick and suffering, is something like one's lost health, former condition, feeling fully alive—for everything to be all right again.

However, Sacks also suggests that the principle underlying adaptation to chronic illness is homeostasis, "achieving the optimum which is possible in (or compossible with) particular circumstances—in short, 'making the best of things' "[19] (p. 234). He argues that optimum health is not some numerical quotient, but the greatest fullness of relationship possible. Diseases thus depart from the optimum by impoverishing, "finite and reductive in mode, endeavoring to reduce the world to itself."[19] (p. 234) Awakening, he then observes, is a rebirth, particularly with a patient with a rich and full self or "inner space" who has been dispossessed by disease. The return of real being and health shows, he argues, that disease is not a thing in itself, but parasitic on health and life and reality. The amazing story of Sacks's patients "awakenings" after decades of being physically and mentally frozen comes with the recognition that after so much of the life and structure of the person has been lost, the potential for health and self can survive. The stages he noted in his "awakened" patients were, following the "awakening," a tribulation, followed by an accommodation.

Sacks's dialectic approach to awakening may be a useful model in which to study not necessarily just the response to protease inhibitor–induced improvement, but the response to disease itself. This will depend on the fullness of relationship that pre-existed the illness, and the degree of richness and fullness of the "inner space" of the person on which, to use Sacks's metaphor, the disease has become a parasite. It will also depend on what it took for the patient to feel fully alive prior to the illness—whether in terms of relationships, control, external contexts, spiritual meaning in life, and so on. Often, however, the meaning of what it meant to be fully alive will not become conscious until it has been lost, and attempts to accommodate this will constitute the center of the adaptation process. Others may be so overwhelmed by the disease that they will become dispossessed by it. We have noted the interesting phraseology used by some people with HIV disease, saying not that "I have HIV," but that "I *am* HIV." Such identification with the aggressor may itself be a provision of meaning in a life or a mode of coping, and an extension of what Sontag[7] sees as the metaphor of AIDS as an invader of not only persons but of society.

Living on the boundary is one consequence of the meanings of HIV and AIDS, which Sontag[7] describes as being something ingenious, unpredictable, and novel, in other words, something for which there is no useful model of how to behave since it is not only new but also constantly changing. Thus, the meaning of living with HIV and AIDS may constantly be in flux in much the same way as the symptoms of the immunodeficiency may vary from person to person, time to time, and place to place. HIV and AIDS have in common with other chronic and potentially terminal illnesses, such as cancers, many of their meanings, adaptations, and coping strategies. However, the meanings ascribed to HIV/AIDS and its very variability set it aside in a psychological sense. Sontag[7] describes it as one of the most meaning-laden of diseases, along with leprosy and syphilis (and thus one of the most stigmatizing). This will become apparent when one examines the richness of the responses of men with HIV disease.

REFERENCES

1. Barnard D. Chronic illness and the dynamics of hoping. In: Toombs SK, Barnard D, Carson RA, eds. *Chronic Illness: From Experience to Policy.* Bloomington: Indiana University Press; 1995; 38–57.
2. Kleinman A. *The Illness Narratives: Suffering, Healing and the Human Condition.* New York: Basic Books; 1988.
3. Murphy RF. *The Body Silent.* New York: Henry Holt; 1987.
4. Taylor SE. Adjustment to threatening events: A theory of cognitive adaptation. *American Psychologist* 1983; 38:1161–1173.
5. Brody H. *Stories of Sickness.* New Haven: Yale University Press; 1987.
6. Sontag S. *Illness as Metaphor.* New York: Farrar, Strauss & Giroux; 1978.
7. Sontag S. *AIDS and Its Metaphors.* New York: Farrar, Strauss & Giroux; 1989.
8. Butler S. *Erewhon.* (1872). New York: Penguin; 1985.
9. Lipowski ZJ. Physical illness, the individual and the coping process. *Psychiatric Medicine* 1970; 1:91–102.
10. Schüssler G. Coping strategies and individual meanings of illness. *Social Science and Medicine* 1992; 34:427–432.
11. Miller SM, Rodoletz M, Schroeder CM, *et al.* Applications of the monitoring process model to coping with severe long-term medical threats. *Health Psychology* 1996; 15:216–225.
12. Ross MW, Tebble WEM, Viliunas D. Staging of psychological reactions to HIV infection in asymptomatic homosexual men. *Journal of Psychology and Human Sexuality* 1989; 2:93–104.
13. Kübler-Ross E. *On Death and Dying.* London: Tavistock; 1970.
14. Cass VC. Homosexual identity formation: A theoretical model. *Journal of Homosexuality* 1979; 4:219–235.
15. Ross MW, Ryan L. The little deaths: Perceptions of HIV, sexuality and quality of life in gay men. *Journal of Psychology and Human Sexuality* 1995; 7:1–20.
16. Greer S, Morris T, Pettingale KW. Psychological responses to breast cancer: effect on outcome. *Lancet* 1979; 2:785–787.

17. Ross MW, Hunter CE, Condon J, *et al.* The Mental Adjustment to HIV Scale: Measurement and dimensions of response to AIDS/HIV disease. *AIDS Care* 1994; 6:407–411.
18. Watson M, Greer S, Bliss JM. *Mental Adjustment to Cancer (MAC) Users' Manual.* Sutton, UK: Institute of Cancer Research; 1989.
19. Sacks O. *Awakenings.* London: Picador; 1991.

3

HIV Testing and Its Impact

Testing for HIV is the first step in the chain of events leading to the discovery that one is HIV seropositive and thus HIV infected. However, reasons for seeking testing, the psychological impact of testing, and disclosure after obtaining a positive HIV test result may all show considerable variation. Indeed, Phillips and Coates,[1] in a review of HIV counseling and testing research and policy issues, note that much of the literature is based on samples of convenience, and that the randomized sample designs that would be required to determine the impact of counseling and testing have not been carried out or may not be ethically appropriate. Much of the research on testing covers populations other than gay and bisexual men—women and children, heterosexual people, and injecting drug users.

In this chapter, we will pay more attention to those studies investigating gay and bisexual men and men who have sex with men. However, a number of studies on HIV testing in heterosexual women and men raise general issues that apply to testing regardless of sexual orientation, or alternatively highlight important differences, and these will also be discussed.

SEEKING HIV TESTING

Seeking testing is the final step of an emotional-cognitive decision-making process. Most people struggle with rational versus emotional forces in the process and the final decision may be more or less difficult to make. However, not all individuals seek testing if they have been at risk of HIV infection, and often people will seek testing without any appreciable risk. In a Canadian study, Myers et al.[2] investigated 1,300 men in gay venues (including bars and bathhouses) in Toronto, and found that only 53% had been tested for HIV, of whom 26% were infected. Predictors of being tested included metropolitan residence, history of anal intercourse, and being in a nonmonogamous relationship or no relationship. Reasons that respondents gave for not being tested included anonymity (fear of being on a government list, negative impact on one's career, negative impact on one's relationship); self-perceived health (probably being negative, being healthy, never knowingly having had sex with an HIV-infected person); and not seeing any benefit in being tested for, or being in denial about, HIV infection (not wanting to know, believing that nothing can be done about HIV infection). Further, of those who believed that they had an almost certain chance or strong chance of having HIV infection, two-thirds had been tested, significantly more than the less than half of those who felt that they had a low chance.

Interestingly, of those who had not previously been tested, one-third indicated that they intended to test, with a further third unsure: whereas 70% of those previously negative and 60% of those previously positive indicated the intention to retest. This suggests a degree of shock, denial, or disbelief about the test result. Those who engaged in anal intercourse, and who were younger, were more likely to take the test.

In a follow-up to this study, Godin et al.[3] found that in 1,500 gay or bisexual men in 125 gay-related venues in Canada the most important variables predicting uptake of testing were having a positive attitude to the test and a higher sense of behavioral control (how easy it was for them to take the test). They speculate that as testing becomes more normative in a region, more people are likely to take it. They also note, however, that the less educated take more tests, and that test taking is unrelated to the risk of the behavior. These data suggest that there may be a subpopulation of men who use repeated tests to reinforce their belief that their previous behavior, even if risky, is not risky if they remain negative. Testing may thus serve the function of providing psychological support for risky behavior.

In a study of HIV testing in a group of 50 heterosexual people in Australia, Lupton, McCarthy, and Chapman[4] note that those who volunteer for testing must identify themselves as at-risk for a fatal and stigmatizing illness for which there is no cure; undergo an uncomfortable medical testing procedure, including a relatively long waiting period for results; publicly admit (to strangers) that they are at-risk for this disease; weigh the societal risks of undergoing the test process; weigh whether they can psychologically navigate a positive result; and return to learn the results of the test. Such acceptance, they note, presupposes a rational thought process, in which people have weighed the likelihood that they may have been exposed, and then taken steps to find out if they are infected and change their behavior accordingly. Lupton, McCarthy, and Chapman report that the most common reason for seeking the test was wanting to know, with the second and third most common reasons respectively being more than one sexual partner in the previous year and having sex with a casual partner before the test. The meanings they report as emerging from qualitative analyses of the reasons for testing included feelings of personal vulnerability and maintenance of bodily integrity and bodily boundaries. The second set of reasons included pressure from partners to find out their serostatus in order to end the necessity for using condoms. In such cases, the HIV test was also a responsible and sensible procedure before entering a long-term sexual relationship, a way of proving one really cared about one's partner and more definitive than a verbal reassurance from the partner of lack of infection. Thus, they argue, the HIV test is important "social currency" (it provides a value to the individual if they are negative) and is seen as congruent with enhanced sexual attractiveness. They see it as part of a "new sexual etiquette" or as a response to ultimatums by partners, usually female partners. Others saw it as serving the function of providing knowledge, like a Papanicolaou ("Pap") smear, despite the fact that there may be limited possibilities for treatment. Thus, testing was contextual rather than related to risk perception—few of their respondents seriously believed that the result would come back positive, despite anxieties between the time of the test and obtaining the result. Thus, for the majority, the HIV testing experience was symbolic and reassuring, especially as the test does not protect against infection or against partner infidelity.

Similar data on decision making in HIV testing was obtained in the United Kingdom in a qualitative study by Coyle, Knapp, and O'Dea.[5] They noted that there is a conceptual difference between those groups who may be sensitized to their risk (e.g., gay men in HIV Pattern 1 countries) and those in low prevalence areas or who do not see themselves at risk. The testing trajectory, they noted, is different for the two groups, with the "low risk" (as self-perceived) group making up their minds well before approaching health professionals and almost always returning for test results, while the data for the "high risk" group show a much greater concern about first taking the test, and then, second, returning for the results. The "low risk" group sought testing for "peace of mind" and relationship issues and recognized (perhaps inappropriately) that the likelihood of an HIV seropositive result was minimal, not having seen themselves at risk of HIV infection until the matter was raised by others. Given the relatively low HIV seroprevalence in Sweden, even among men who have sex with men, it may be that the "low risk" model may be as useful as the U.S.-based models of testing in gay men. Coyle, Knapp, and O'Dea suggest that there are four main reasons for having an HIV test: first, a belief that the person could have been exposed to HIV based on an acknowledgment of past risk behavior; second, a desire for reassurance and for relief of the psychological stress associated with not knowing one's HIV status; third, reasons related to present or future decision making about health, reproduction, and sexual practices; and fourth, advice to take the test by health professionals or friends. It is worth noting that relief of the stress associated with not knowing one's HIV status may be occasioned by a positive as well as a negative test result. The data suggest that the decision to take a test may be based both on risk perception and on potential (and previous) coping mechanisms with negative life events.

Rates of return for testing in gay men may be low, even where the test is offered free. In a 1988 study in small towns in Pennsylvania, Silvestre et al.[6] studied over 100 men who were offered HIV testing. Only half of the men who volunteered accepted testing, and only 17% of the total sample returned for their test results, despite an educational session and several invitations to return for test results. Those who did *not* accept testing were more likely to be better educated and of racial or ethnic minorities. Similarly, those who did not return for test results were also more likely to be better educated. In terms of acculturation into the gay community, those men who read gay magazines or newspapers were more likely to refuse testing than nonreaders; however, they were also more likely, if tested, to return for results. Members of gay organizations were more likely to refuse HIV testing; similarly, though, if tested, they were more likely to return for results. Results of a logistic regression analysis indicated that men with a bachelor's degree were three times more likely to refuse testing, and that readers of gay magazines were also three times as likely to refuse testing. Race and ethnicity as a predictor disappeared in this multivariate analysis. Men with a university degree were twice as likely not to return for results if tested. These data illustrate that the better educated, from both the conventional perspective and in terms of HIV from their acculturation in the gay community and readership of gay print media, preferred not to know their HIV serostatus. This is probably a logical approach given that at the time of the study, there was no effective intervention to prevent the progression of HIV disease. Not knowing was at the time an effective coping mechanism, akin to avoidance and denial.

Access to HIV testing is also a consideration in who gets tested. Henrickson[7] reports on the success of an outreach HIV van in Connecticut, where users of the van that parked in their neighborhoods was 95% African American or Latino, and 60% injecting drug users. Rates of HIV infection in this new population were 27%, five times higher than in the primary clinic site. However, the rate of return for test results was only 20% for the van, compared with nearly three-quarters for the primary clinic site. These data suggest that access to testing, as much as intention, may influence testing rates.

Differences are also apparent in reasons for testing of those attending anonymous testing centers and the general population. A combined clinic and telephone survey methodology study in Switzerland[8] found that the distribution of the client characteristic were not different, but that the reasons for testing differed significantly between sites. Those in the anonymous clinics were more likely to be tested at the suggestion of friends or partners, and nearly half reported a new regular sexual partner in the past year. In contrast, those in the general population were more likely to have been tested at the suggestion of their physician. These two studies illustrate some of the differences in access or perceived access to health care (including HIV testing) between the United States and Europe.

PSYCHOLOGICAL RESPONSES TO HIV SEROCONVERSION

The waiting period of the test result is usually perceived as stressful. Some describe it as almost unbearable, filled with worries and horrifying fantasies but also in terms of emotional numbness.[9] The immediate reactions to an HIV-seropositive diagnosis can indeed be expressed in a diversity of ways; from shock, chaos, aggressiveness to grief, hopelessness, sadness, and anxiety to confirmation and "relief."[9–11] To psychologically protect oneself from the strong, painful, and overwhelming emotions related to the HIV status disclosure, the individual may make use of various defense mechanisms, such as emotional numbness, denial, and repression.

The psychological well-being correlates of HIV status disclosure have been described by Ostrow et al.[12] in a Chicago sample as being a significantly adverse one in those who learned they were seropositive, and a positive effect of learning one is seronegative. Ostrow et al. were able to disentangle the effect of impact by comparing those who had asked for their HIV test results to be disclosed to them with those who did not want to know their results. Reasons for requesting disclosure included concern as to whether they had been exposed to HIV in previous sexual activities, desire for information about their future health, and concern about exposing sexual partners. Interestingly, 95% of seropositive men and 66% of seronegative men correctly guessed their HIV antibody status, although those who were HIV seropositive reported significantly more symptoms. Ostrow et al. also noted that all their groups showed a significant reduction in sexual risk behavior.

On all the dimensions measured (somatization, obsessive-compulsive symptoms, interpersonal difficulties, depression, anxiety, and well-being), those who were HIV seropositive scored significantly worse after disclosure compared with before. In contrast, the nondisclosed HIV seropositive men generally showed improved psychological well-being over time. For the HIV seronegative men, both disclosed and nondisclosed subjects showed the same trend toward improvement over time. Clearly, psychological maladjustment and psychological symptoms increase significantly for those who have a disclosed HIV infection, compared with controls who are not disclosed, and with those uninfected, whether their HIV antibody status has been disclosed to them or not.

In a similar study, Perry et al.[13] evaluated over 200 asymptomatic adults in New York before HIV test notification, after notification, and two and ten weeks later. For the HIV seronegatives, immediately after notification there were decreases in several measures of anxiety and depression, fears of getting AIDS, and of having infected others, which were sustained on follow-up. Interestingly, for the HIV seropositive subjects, immediately after notification there were no significant increases in anxiety or depression (although they remained at pretest levels, which were not significantly different from those in the seronegative group before obtaining the test results), and the levels significantly decreased compared with baseline by ten weeks after notification. Nor were the results worse for those HIV seropositives who had predicted that they would be HIV seronegative. The differences in the results of Ostrow et al. and Perry et al., both studies that used predominantly homosexual male samples, suggest that there may be variables other than just the disclosure of seropositive and seronegative HIV results operating.

The response to HIV infection is clearly a dynamic one: indeed, description of the changes over time in response to HIV disease is the central theme of this book. Asymptomatic people who have tested seropositive for HIV go through a series of stages of coping with the disease (although as with all stage models, not all stages need be followed consecutively, and some may be missed). Ross, Tebble, and Viliunas's[14] model of response to HIV infection on clinical observations and interviews with gay men with HIV has already been described in Chapter 2 and is relevant to understanding response to testing seropositive.

Given the incidence of distress following HIV testing in which the result is positive, the question is raised as to whether there are any interventions that might minimize such stress. Perry et al.[15] compared three interventions: standard counseling, a three-session interactive video program including reframing and relaxation techniques, along with educational material, and a six-session individual stress prevention training program. The latter program was based on a stress-innoculation approach, along with cognitive-behavioral treatment for depression, stress, and anxiety. The brief stress reduction program significantly reduced depression, global severity of psychiatric symptoms, and anxiety compared with the other two interventions, in which there was no significant reduction. HIV seronegative subjects experienced a reduction of distress on all three conditions. These data suggest that the distress of receiving an HIV seropositive diagnosis can be reduced by standard stress management techniques.

COMPARISON WITH CANCER DIAGNOSIS

It is difficult to draw direct comparisons between diagnosis with a potentially fatal illness like a cancer and HIV for several reasons. Chief among these is the fact that there is a large degree of uncertainty about the probability of many cancers being fatal or curable, whereas at least until recently, HIV disease was seen as leading to death, although with an uncertain time frame. Cancer is seen as being akin to a lottery. Further, the possibility of infecting others and the knowledge that one was infected by someone else as occurs in HIV/AIDS has little equivalence in cancer, with the exception of cervical cancer, caused in most cases by infection with the genital wart-causing human papillomavirus. While in genital cancers there may be concern about sexual behavior, this is common in HIV infections. And in cancer, with some exceptions, the age group infected is significantly older on average than those infected with HIV. Nevertheless, the literature suggests that there are more similarities than differences in the response, as already noted in Chapter 2.

There is a substantial literature on coping and response to cancer, and only a few studies will be used to illustrate some of the similarities with response to news about HIV infection. Scott, Oberst, and Bookbinder[16] used a longitudinal study design in men with chronic genitourinary cancer and measured stress and anxiety levels immediately before, and six to eight weeks after, biopsies by cystoscopy. In subjects with negative biopsy results, anxiety levels and critical thinking ability were not significantly different before the test procedure than after. Subjects with higher concurrent life stress had higher state anxiety and achieved less resolution of problems. The high anxiety group had more severe behavioral responses, including depression, helplessness, and the inability to set priorities. While the initial diagnosis of cancer had already been made in this group and the diagnostic procedures were used to see if the cancer had recurred, the behavioral responses were similar to those reported in people with positive HIV tests, particularly for those with already existing life stressors. The interaction with existing life stressors is important to note.

In a similar study[17] looking at another genital cancer, cervical Papanicolaou smears to detect precancerous changes in minority women in the United States were carried out. Comparing those women who had had a positive or a negative test result three months after their initial test results, the women with the positive test results showed significant elevations in worries about cancer, and impairments in mood, daily activities, sexual interest, and sleep patterns. These results were most pronounced among women who did not comply with the request to have colposcopy (a further diagnostic and treatment procedure to remove the precancerous tissue). It is unclear whether the distress lead to the decision not to have colposcopy, or whether the decision not to have this treatment caused the distress. The authors suggest that targeting the most vulnerable individuals may reduce distress.

This point is emphasised by Fawzy et al.,[18] looking at an intervention to change the levels of disturbance and improve coping in postsurgical patients with malignant melanoma (an aggressive skin cancer). Their intervention, which consisted of health education, enhancement of problem-solving skills, stress management (relaxation techniques), and psychological support, enabled an improvement to be demonstrated in the intervention group. Specifically, this group showed more vigor and better use of active behavioral coping than the control group. These differences were even more pronounced at six months, suggesting that early intervention will have a major long-term effect. At six months, the intervention produced lower fatigue, confusion, and depression and less overall mood disturbance. This group, while not strictly comparable to the HIV positive group, nevertheless illustrates as in the HIV literature that the negative impact of a potentially life-threatening illness can be successfully ameliorated by brief psychological interventions, and that the distress related to such a diagnosis is similar.

Essentially, any major life-threatening diagnosis will produce reactions characterized by helplessness, depression, denial, and mood disturbance. If it is associated with the genitals, then loss of sexual interest may also result. However, where the group in which the diagnosis occurs is socially stigmatized or discriminated against, the impact of the diagnosis is likely to be magnified. Ross[19] looked at the impact of negative life events in gay men in Australia, and found that their impact on psychological well-being was significantly greater than the impact of similar life events in presumed heterosexual samples. Thus, the more socially stigmatized the group, the stronger the relationship between life events and depression, anxiety, somatic symptoms, and social dysfunction. Ross also noted that those nonhomosexually related items, concerning work and finances, also impacted the psychological adjustment of homosexual men. Thus, an HIV diagnosis that also impacts the potential or actual work, career, and finances of gay men will also impact, indirectly, their psychological well-being, and stigmatization will magnify the effect of an HIV diagnosis.

EFFECT OF HIV TESTING ON SEXUAL BEHAVIOR

The effect of testing, note Phillips and Coates,[1] appears to differ between those who test HIV seropositive and those who test HIV seronegative. Generally, the impact of HIV testing is greater in those who test HIV seropositive. Zenilman et al.[20] matched people by age, sex, and month of test and compared HIV seropositive and seronegative respondents in Baltimore, and observed their return to the STD (sexually transmissible diseases) clinic over time periods up to two years. Seventy-one percent of the HIV infected and 63% of the HIV uninfected people returned for their test results. Of the infected population, 3.9% returned with an STD, significantly less that the uninfected population (10.2%). STD-infected partners were reported by 1.5% of the HIV infected, compared with 3.3% of the uninfected, patients. Age, sexual orientation, and substance use did not predict return with an STD or with contact with an STD-infected partner. These prospective data confirm that an HIV-seropositive result reduces risky sexual behavior compared to receiving an HIV-seronegative result.

In a study of 600 people in Thailand, Müller et al.[21] also found that sexual risk behaviors in people who were HIV infected were significantly lower than in those uninfected. Those who were HIV infected abstained from sex 42% of the time compared with only 14% of the time for the uninfected, and in their past three sexual encounters, the proportions were 44% to 14% for the same groups. Of concern was the fact that only 11% of all participants (14% of married participants) knew the HIV serostatus of their steady partners. However, even the amount of behavior change over time in people who test HIV seropositive is not necessarily high: Landis, Earp, and Koch,[22] in a study in North Carolina, interviewed people on HIV testing and again a year later. Only 24% returned for the interview, and the returnees were more likely to be homosexual men, and more likely to use condoms (48% versus 10% of nonreturners). However, it was disturbing to note that the returnees used condoms *less* than at the baseline interview, suggesting that long-term behavior change is not necessarily common or consistent.

In a Swedish study, Lagergren et al.[23] collected data from 25 clinics over the country and reported that 25% of the population aged 16 to 44 were tested for HIV (half for the purposes of blood donation). All tests were voluntary apart from contacts of people with HIV. HIV prevalence was low: in 1987, only 67 of 79,000 tests were HIV seropositive (4% in homosexual men). There was a significantly higher participation rate in homosexual and bisexual men, including recurrent testing and continued risky sexual behavior. As in previous studies, it was suggested that people may be testing to confirm that the risk behavior did not lead to HIV infection, but that the risk did not deter them from risky behavior.

Available empirical data clearly demonstrate that men who have sex with men in general have made considerable modifications in their sexual repertoires[24] However, empirical findings are contradictory in regard to the impact of HIV-serostatus knowledge on changes of sexual risky behaviors. Several studies[25–29] indicate that those men who are HIV seropositive are less likely to engage in unprotected anal sex than those who are HIV negative or untested. Joseph et al.'s[30] findings are the opposite; men who are HIV negative more often practice protected anal sex than those who are HIV seropositive. Difficulties in maintaining protected sex over time are also reported.[31–34]

Data on the impact of testing itself on sexual behavioral changes are also inconsistent. Various studies have not found any differences between tested and untested gay men.[35–37] Roffman et al.[38] on the other hand did find differences. In a major study of 16 small communities (<180,000 population) across four regions of the United States, they found that 28% had engaged in unprotected anal intercourse in the past two months, and of these, 84% were not protected by engaging in this risk in the context of a monogamous relationship. However, there was a consistent finding at both the individual and community levels of analysis that while those who had been tested had a higher level of sexual activity compared with those who had not been tested, they were also more likely to be engaging in safer sex (as measured by protected oral and anal intercourse). This difference was unchanged when HIV-seropositive men were removed from the analysis. At the city level of analysis, there was a relationship between the proportion of men tested in each city (range 56–81%) and the proportion of men having safer sex (range 9–41%), with the cities where more men had been tested having the highest proportion of men engaging in safer sex. Roffman et al.'s data suggest that testing at a community level does impact sexual safety in a positive way, at least for gay men.

The question as to whether it is the testing or the counseling that provides the impact is difficult to resolve without being able to randomly assign people to testing, counseling, both, or neither, which would be ethically unacceptable. However, Ross[39] was able to compare gay men who had had combined counseling and testing, just testing, just counseling, or neither. He found that the impact on sexual behavior of testing alone and combined counseling and testing was not significantly different, although significantly better than counseling alone or neither counseling nor testing. These data suggest that the impact of having the test (or the type of person who decides to have the test, as suggested by Roffman et al.'s data) is related to a reduction in sexual risk behavior.

SELF-DISCLOSURE OF SEROSTATUS

Self-disclosure relates to the degree of the individual's openness about his HIV status within his social network and toward his past, current, and potential sexual partners. According to Mansergh et al., as quoted by Holt et al.,[40] disclosure increases with time from diagnosis and with an increase in symptoms. It is also evident that disclosure is more likely to occur with significant others than to less significant ones.[41]

As noted in the work of Müller et al.[21] in Thailand, disclosure of HIV serostatus may not be common or consistent. Similar findings are found among gay men. Recent studies[42,43] suggest that gay men with HIV often do not disclose their status to their sexual partners. Klitzman's study[44] revealed a variety of patterns of self-disclosure. Different standards of disclosure were often followed contingent on the type of sexual partner. Further data showed that disclosure was often indirect or ambiguous and responsibility was often deferred to the other partner.

Data from Western countries suggest that figures for disclosure of serostatus, while considerably higher for gay men, are nevertheless short of adequate even after repeated interventions. In a study of nearly 130 HIV-infected adults, Perry et al.[45] reported counseling every six months, up to a period of 2.3 years. Patients after counseling had told 77% of present steady sexual partners and 42% of present casual sexual partners, and similarly 70% of past steady sexual partners and 47% of past casual sexual partners. However, a third had still not informed *any* of their sexual partners, past or present. Nondisclosers were more likely to have lower social support and higher discomfort about their sexual orientation. In a related study in San Francisco, Stempel, Moulton, and Moss[46] found that after one year, HIV-seropositive gay and bisexual men had told 92% of their gay friends, 82% of their primary partners, 56% of new sexual partners, 46% of co-workers, 71% of their physicians, 37% of their dentists, 57% of their psychotherapists, and 37% of family members. They reported the most negative reactions from male family members and primary sexual partners. Even in a city with such a large gay population and openness about HIV issues, given the high HIV-seroprevalence rate, the lack of disclosure (only about half of new sexual partners) is a cause for concern. Respondents reported that the major issues precluding disclosure were fears of stigmatization (61% at baseline, falling to 36% after one year).

SUMMARY

Taken together, these data show that reasons for seeking testing and for disclosure vary. Further HIV testing will affect both sexual behavior and psychological functioning and coping in gay men, and the influence of testing is similar to the impact of some cancer-related diagnoses. However, the research also suggests that given related issues of stigmatization, discrimination, possible lack of social support, and the uncertainty of disease progression, the impact of the HIV test, if it is seropositive, will have ramifications far beyond the time surrounding the test and the delivery of the result.

REFERENCES

1. Phillips KA, Coates TJ. HIV counseling and testing: Research and policy issues. *AIDS Care* 1995; 7:115–124.
2. Myers T, Orr KW, Locker D, *et al.* Factors affecting gay and bisexual men's decisions and intentions to seek HIV testing. *American Journal of Public Health* 1993; 83:701–704.
3. Godin G, Myers T, Lambert J, *et al.* Understanding the intention of gay and bisexual men to take the HIV antibody test. *AIDS Education and Prevention* 1997; 9:31–41.
4. Lupton D, McCarthy S, Chapman S. "Doing the right thing": the symbolic meanings and experiences of having an HIV antibody test. *Social Science and Medicine* 1995; 41:173–180.
5. Coyle A, Knapp M, O'Dea E. Decision making in HIV testing among a group with low HIV risk. *Journal of Evaluation in Clinical Practice* 1996; 2:223–230.
6. Silvestre AJ, Kingsley LA, Rinaldo C, *et al.* Factors associated with participation in HIV antibody screening and results is closure. *Health and Social Work* 1993; 18:248–258.
7. Henrickson M. A mobile HIV education, counseling and testing unit: a pilot initiative. *AIDS Education and Prevention* 1990; 2:137–144.
8. Rossi I, Jeannin A, Dubois-Arber F, *et al.* Comparison of the clientele of an anonymous HIV test centre and persons tested in the general population. *AIDS Care* 1998; 10:89–103.
9. Nilsson Schönnesson L. HIV infection: Trauma, psychic metabolism, and psychological well-being. A study of 29 Swedish gay HIV-positive men. Unpublished research report (in Swedish). Stockholm; 1993.
10. Kaisch K, Anton-Culver H. Psychological and social consequences of HIV exposure: Homosexuals in Southern California. *Psychology and Health* 1989; 3:63–75.
11. Hoffman MA. Counseling the HIV-infected client: A psychosocial model for assessment and intervention. *The Counseling Psychologist* 1991; 9(4):467–542.
12. Ostrow DG, Joseph JG, Kessler R, *et al.* Disclosure of HIV antibody status: behavioral and mental health correlates. *AIDS Education and Prevention* 1989; 1:1–11.
13. Perry SW, Jacobsberg LB, Fishman B, *et al.* Psychological responses to serological testing for HIV. *AIDS* 1990; 4:145–152.
14. Ross MW, Tebble WEM, Viliunas D. Staging of psychological reactions to HIV infection in asymptomatic homosexual men. *Journal of Psychology and Human Sexuality* 1989; 2:93–104.
15. Perry S, Fishman B, Jacobsberg L, *et al.* Effectiveness of psychoeducational interventions in reducing emotional distress after Human Immunodeficiency Virus antibody testing. *Archives of General Psychiatry* 1991; 48:143–147.

16. Scott DW, Oberst MT, Bookbinder MI. Stress-coping response to genitourinary carcinoma in men. *Nursing Research* 1984; 33:325–329.
17. Lerman C, Miller SM, Scarborough R, *et al.* Adverse psychologic consequences of positive cytologic cervical screening. *American Journal of Obstetrics and Gynecology* 1991; 165:658–662.
18. Fawzy FI, Cousins N, Fawzy NW, *et al.* A structured psychiatric intervention for cancer patients. Changes over time in methods of coping and affective disturbance. *Archives of General Psychiatry* 1990; 47:720–725.
19. Ross MW. The relationship between the vents and mental health in homosexual men. *Journal of Clinical Psychology* 1990; 46:402–411.
20. Zenilman JM, Erickson B, Fox R, *et al.* Effect of HIV posttest counseling on STD incidence. *Journal of the American Medical Association* 1992; 267:843–845.
21. Müller O, Sarangbin S, Ruxrungtham K, *et al.* Sexual risk behavior reduction associated with voluntary HIV counseling and testing in HIV infected patients in Thailand. *AIDS Care* 1995; 7:567–572.
22. Landis SE, Earp JL, Koch GG. Impact of HIV testing and counseling on subsequent sexual behavior. *AIDS Education and Prevention* 1992; 4:61–70.
23. Lagergren M, Giesecke J, Hallqvist J, *et al.* Anonymous inquiries in Sweden regarding the individual's motives for HIV antibody testing. *AIDS Education and Prevention* 1990; 2:171–180.
24. Nilsson Schönnesson L, Dolezal C. HIV-related risk factors among Swedish gay men. *Scandinavian Journal of Sexology* 1998; 1(1):51–62.
25. Exner TM, Dolezal CL, Liu X, *et al.* Sexual risk behavior in the course of HIV disease: HIV+ and HIV− gay men. Poster at the International Academy of Sex Research, 21st Annual Meeting, Provincetown, MA, September 20–24, 1995.
26. Schechter M, Craib K, Willoughby B, *et al.* Patterns of sexual behavior and condom use in a cohort of homosexual men. *American Journal of Public Health* 1988; 78:1535–1538.
27. Coates TJ, Morin SF, McKusick L. Behavioral consequences of AIDS antibody testing among gay men. *Journal of the American Medical Association* 1987; 258:1889.
28. Fox R, Odaka NJ, Brookmeyer R, *et al.*. Effect of antibody test disclosure on subsequent sexual activity in homosexual men. *AIDS* 1987; 1:241–246.
29. Catania JA, Coates TJ, Stall R, *et al.* Changes in condom use among homosexual men in San Francisco. *Health Psychology* 1991; 10(3):190–199.
30. Joseph JG, Montgomery SB, Kessler RC, *et al.* Behavioral risk-reduction in a cohort of homosexual men: Two-year follow-up. Third International Conference on AIDS, Washington DC, USA; 1987.
31. McCusker J, Stoddard M, McDonald M, *et al.*. Maintenance of behavioral change in a cohort of homosexually active men. *AIDS*, 1992; 6:861–868.
32. Hart G, Boulton M, Fitzpatrick R. "Relapse" to unsafe sexual behavior among gay men: A critique of recent behavioral HIV/AIDS research. *Sociology of Health and Illness* 1991; 4(2):216–232.
33. Adib M, Joseph JG, Ostrow DG. Relapse in safer sexual practices among homosexual men: Two-year follow-up from the Chicago–MACS/ccs. *AIDS* 1990; 5(6):757–760.
34. Stall RD, Ekstrand MI, Pollack I, *et al.* Relapse from safer sex: The next challenge for AIDS prevention efforts. *Journal of Acquired Immune Deficiency Syndrome* 1990; 3:1181–1187.
35. Detels R, English P, Visscher B, *et al.* Seroconversion, sexual activity, and condom use among 2915 HIV seronegative men followed for up to 2 years. *Journal of Acquired Immune Deficiency Syndromes* 1989; 2:77–83.
36. Ginzburg H, Fleming P, Miller K. Selected public health observations derived from the Multicenter AIDS cohort study. *Journal of Acquired Immune Deficiency Syndromes* 1988; 1:2–7.
37. Calabrese LH, Buck H, Easley KA. Persistence of high risk sexual activity among homosexual men in an area of low incidence for acquired immunodeficiency syndrome. *AIDS Research* 1986; 2:357–361.

38. Roffman RA, Kalichman SC, Kelly JA, *et al.* HIV antibody testing of gay men in smaller US cities. *AIDS Care* 1995; 7:405–413.
39. Ross MW. Relationship of combinations of AIDS counseling and testing to safer sex and condom use in homosexual men. *Community Health Studies* 1988; 12:322–327.
40. Holt R, Court P, Vedhara K, *et al.* The role of disclosure in coping with HIV infection. *AIDS Care* 1998; 10(1):49–60.
41. Hays RB, McKusick L, Pollak L, *et al.* Disclosing HIV seropositivity to significant others. *AIDS* 1993; 7:425–431.
42. Perry SW, Ryan J, Fogel K, *et al.* Voluntarily informing others of positive HIV test results. Patterns of notification by infected gay men. *Hospital Community Psychiatry* 1990; 41:549–551.
43. Marks G, Richardson J, Maldonado N. Self-disclosure of HIV infection to sexual partners. *American Journal of Public Health* 1991; 81:1321–1322.
44. Klitzman R. Adapting to HIV: Narratives of illness and psychological health and behavior. Abst. First international conference on biopsychosocial aspects of HIV-infection. Amsterdam, The Netherlands; 1991.
45. Perry SW, Card CAL, Moffatt M, *et al.* Self-disclosure of HIV infection to sexual partners after repeated counseling. *AIDS Education and Prevention* 1994; 6:403–411.
46. Stempel RR, Moulton JM, Moss AR. Self-disclosure of HIV antibody test results; The San Francisco General Hospital cohort. *AIDS Education and Prevention* 1995; 7:116–123.

4

HIV-Related Threats

The person living with HIV is not only confronted with the HIV diagnosis as such but also to various physical, social, and sexual threats toward his physical, social, and sexual existence throughout the disease process. In this chapter we describe each of the threats and illuminate them by empirical data from other studies and the quantitative and qualitative analysis of Dr. Schönnesson's psychotherapeutic notes of gay men with HIV.

The diagnosis of HIV infection is regarded as a traumatic event. Traumatic events and experiences are, according to Hacking,[1] "wounds to the spirit." Whereas Freud described trauma as almost always somebody doing something, that is, an intentional act, Janet (as cited in Hacking[1]) viewed the trauma itself not as a human action but as an event or a state. It should be emphasized though that from a theoretical perspective it takes an appraisal process[2] to determine whether HIV infection is indeed traumatic to the individual. However, we start from the basic assumption that HIV is a trauma in that it is "out of the ordinary"[3] (p. 53) and is experienced as a threat to survival and self-preservation. and is "markedly distressing to almost anyone."[4] The core of the trauma is its basic survival threat or in Lifton's[5] wording, a "death imprint." Fischer and Riedesser (quoted in Hammelstein[6]) maintain that the specific traumatic feature of HIV is caused by its internal threatening influence. "Thus, the 'traumatic reaction' is characterized by the paradox that one wants to flee from something which lies within, in the interior of the psychophysical self-relationship, and which is not avoidable"[6] (p. 375). HIV is also a traumatic event in that the individual is confronted with various threats or stressors that may draw the individual into a realm of hopelessness and powerlessness.

PHYSICAL THREATS

HIV as a Threat to Our Physical Survival

The individual's physical survival is abruptly challenged by the diagnosis of HIV, and his life is disrupted in that it penetrates into the immune system, blood, and the semen. These vital fluids also have a symbolic meaning of life. Blood is the symbol of feeling alive, passionate, being inextricably connected. Semen represents life and its continuity and the immune system the protection of life. The infection illuminates our fragility as human beings and life's finitude through death, the one certainty of our lives: "Our own survival ... becomes seriously questioned."[7] On the other hand, the tragedy of death is a precondition of human life. "But because we will die we try to live as if we were immortal, as if we had an eternity to fulfil our lives' tasks"[7] (p. 160).

Enormous progress in medical treatment has over the years accomplished to manage and postpone HIV-related symptoms and diseases, but the infection as such is still not curable. First came AZT, then Videx, Hivid, and Epivir, and most recently protease inhibitors and combination therapies. The latter arouse hope but also cautiousness and even skepticism among people with HIV. Although protease inhibitors (e.g., Viracept, Crixivan, Invirase, Norvir, and Fortovase) appear to provide much benefit, we still do not know about their long-term benefits, side effects, development of resistance, or the psychological impact when the new medication works only for a short time or does not work at all.

Life expectancy for people with HIV is, however, much longer today than a decade ago. In 1994 a new concept was introduced at the international AIDS conference, that of "long-term nonprogressor." It refers to people whose HIV seropositive serostatus has been established unequivocably yet who remain immunologically healthy and physically asymptomatic for 12 years or longer.[8] The time span has also changed with respect to survival after being diagnosed with AIDS. In the early 1980s gay men with HIV were in general told they would live, at the most, another year or two. As a consequence of the perceived "death sentence," some of them decided to quit their jobs in favor of disability or sick leave. As Benny comments:

> I would anyway die in a very short time, and I really wanted to get the best out of my life. I wanted to fullfil my dreams such as traveling around the world.

They said their goodbyes and they adjusted to a "death orientation, prepared to give up their life."[9] But quite a few of these men have remained quite healthy over the years (i.e., long-term nonprogressors), and today they regret their decision years ago. As Leonard says:

> Today I am angry that I left work. Now it is almost impossible to get back into the labor market. And how am I to explain why I haven't had a job for eight years?

Others express disappointment that life did not turn out the way they had expected. George and Frank make similar points, respectively:

> Death cheated me.

> Well, I took a bank loan in order to go around the world—thinking that I didn't have to worry about paying it back, as I would soon be dead. And here I am—still alive! And the loan is also there but now even higher because of the interest.

To some people it is more or less a burden to be a "long-term survivor" or a "long-term nonprogressor." Gerald and Brett express this in different ways, respectively:

> This waiting to become sick and to die is so terribly wasting.
>
> I think it is a mystery why I am still alive. I don't even have a real symptom. I don't understand why I am still here on earth whereas so many of my friends have died.

The latter statement reflects feelings of survivor guilt that are quite commonly presented in clinical practice. The men compare themselves with friends that became infected at the same time or subsequently and now are dead or very sick. Survival guilt stems from the randomness of the situation, the fact that survival or death may be largely a matter of caprice, fate, or luck. Within the survival guilt context it is imperative to remember that living in the gay subcultures that have been so heavily struck by AIDS takes its toll in terms of multiple loss. As a result of being confronted with these "dying systems" many gay men have on an individual as well as on a communal level become alienated from a life orientation and suffer from survival guilt.

In 1996 the treatment of HIV disease changed dramatically in that triple "combination therapy" became the new standard of treatment. A psychological consequence of this change is that those gay men who are long-term nonprogressors or long-term survivors are facing another form of survival issue that is related to the future. Bill has known his serostatus for 11 years. His life goal a decade ago was to "take advantage" of his short life expectancy. He calculated that he would be dead before his thirty-fifth birthday. Bill has passed that date by five years. These years have from time to time been a dread to him: "I have been waiting and waiting for symptoms to develop but in vain." He has now been offered, and accepted, the new combination therapy. During one session he talks about his doubts about the medication. He finds his life getting more and more circumscribed because of the tough medical regime. So far, he has not noticed any physical side effects but suffers from psychological effects:

> There is that strange feeling coming over me. Does this new medication mean that I will have to live until I am 60 or even 70 years old? I don't know if I would like that to happen. I have never seen, not before HIV either, that aging as a gay should be an option.

This new situation—to be "offered" a life perspective—that Bill shares with many gay men means that their "death-oriented" life attitude is challenged. Paradoxically as it may sound, a potential life perspective can also induce life anxiety. Some[10,11] have raised the question whether gay men, who are long-term nonprogressor/survivors, are ready to face life again.

Regardless of being a long-term nonprogressor or long-term survivor or not, people with HIV must live with various physical threats. These include stressors such as uncertainty and worries about the disease progression and its potential patterns of HIV-related symptoms and diseases as well as treatment concerns. One study[12] among asymptomatic gay men showed that those men who reported intrusive HIV thoughts also experienced depressive or anxious AIDS stress, strong worries about becoming sick, and that they ran a higher risk than others of developing HIV-related symptoms and diseases.

Table 1. Meanings of Physical Treats over the Four HIV Disease Phases

The asymptomatic phase	The mild symptomatic phase	The severe symptomatic phase	The terminal phase
Time;	Bewilderment;	Fear;	Confirmation;
Worries about progression;	Uncertainty;	To loose control;	Loosing control;
	HIV becomes a reality;	Body deterioration;	"Enough is enough"
Time-concerns	Healthy-sick?	Progression	

The quantitative analysis of the psychotherapeutic notes showed that all the men were engaged in worries and concerns related to HIV. Although fewer men in the course of the disease process brought up HIV-related concerns, the intensity with which they were talked about significantly increased over the disease phases. The qualitative analysis implied that the meaning of physical threats changed over the disease process, as illustrated in Table 1. Each of the meanings is described and highlighted with quotes from the gay men.

In the asymptomatic stage the men expressed worries and time-oriented concern about progression. The men asked themselves *when* they would get sick: "How long do I have to wait?" They were also concerned about what kind of symptoms they might develop. The most feared symptom was "that HIV will attack my brain." It is very clear from the quotes that the men struggled with uncertainty about their physical future.

In the following phase, the mild symptomatic one, worries were expressed in terms of uncertainty. "The uncertainty is so exhausting." To some HIV "becomes a reality" in this phase. Stephen says:

> When I got my first symptoms, well then I realized in my guts that something was wrong with me. Then all of a sudden I felt my life threatened.

Others started to ask themselves whether they should keep fighting or just give in to HIV. Questions related to whether one is sick or healthy were also raised. Nicholas, for example, asks: "OK I have these minor dermatological symptoms, but that's all. I am doing fine. But I don't know if I am sick or?" Similarly, Adam asks: "When should I define myself as ill?"

Others had the experience that they were placed into the "sick role" despite the fact they perceived themselves as healthy. Roger observes: "I hate the way they (his colleagues) pamper me and symbolically pat me on my head. They do it because I am HIV-positive."

Peter describes how he experiences his friends:

> They almost seem to be disappointed or at least very skeptical when I say I am doing fine. It is as though I'm not supposed to be fine as I'm HIV positive.

These quotes reflect bewilderment as to one's role within the HIV realm—sick or healthy. There also seems to be a dilemma around who is the one to define when the person is sick or healthy; the person himself (subjective health/disease) or the physician/social network (the "objective" standpoint). As we know from other serious diseases these two "definitions" are not necessarily congruent. Another aspect of the "sick-healthy" role, which leads to uncertainty, is medication. Adam, whose CD-4 (T-helper cells) counts had begun to fall, got very confused when his doctor brought up discussion about AZT.

> Well, my doctor says I'm healthy, so why should I then take AZT? AZT is only given to people who are really sick—and I am not sick. Or am I sick? This doesn't make sense to me.

Medication issues, regardless of disease phase, were discussed and reflected upon by the vast majority of the men. Medications are also a reminder of having HIV: "There is no way out now." "This is the beginning of the end" or in Klitzman's[13] words, people "are forced against their will to incorporate the possibility of death into their lives."

The meaning of the physical threats changed into fear about current and potential bodily deterioration in the third phase (the severe symptomatic phase). Steven for example got very frightened when he realized that his digital watch did not make any sense to him: "What does 2:13 P.M. actually mean?" Charles expressed his fear as to cytomegalovirus (CMV): "Do you think CMV is starting up its battle now?" It is common in this phase that the men also shared their fear to lose control over their lives because of the disease, as expressed in Frank's words, "I'm like a whirling leaf in the wind."

Another characteristic of the severe symptomatic phase is medical crises interspersed with periods of good or relatively good health. Many people with HIV describe the situation as a roller coaster and a flip-flopping between crisis and normalcy, life and death.[13]

Those fears that were expressed in the third phase of the disease were confirmed in the final phase in that they became reality, and many men expressed a sense of "enough is enough."

HIV as a Threat to Our Psychological Survival

HIV threatens not only our physical but also our psychological survival. In other words, there are two sides of our existence—body and the self. Kierkegaard[14] argues that it looks like some kind of hoax that we can have consciousness, deep feelings, and self-expression, yet also be creatures that die.

The reason why threats to our physical existence also threaten our psychological survival is a consequence of the close link between the body and the development of our self-concept. From a psychodynamic perspective, the conception of one's own body plays a crucial role in the development of our selves and construction of reality. The discovery of one's own body and eventually the development of one's body image occur through memories of internal sensations but also external sensations and experiences in interplay with others. The body image is the nucleus of the self, which is reflected in these quotes by William and David, respectively:

> My body is me.

> I have great confidence in my body and that means that I have confidence in myself.

Consequently, the body is also important to self-image and self-esteem. In extension it means that when HIV attacks the body not only fear of physical death is evoked but also fears about losing one's sense of body boundaries, one's self, and ultimately dying psychologically.

In sharp contrast to the "ill" body stands the strong Western societal emphasis in recent years on the "perfect" body, physical fitness, and health. This is a paradox. On the one hand we do know that our body must decay and does so. But at the same time we make a pact with our body (by means of healthy living) not to let us down. In that way, Weeks[7] argues, the body becomes the locus for our avoidance of death. The "perfect body" serves, in other words, as a defense against death fear.

Our bodies also play an important role in our strivings to be affirmed and acknowledged as a sexual person. People with HIV may experience their sexual self-esteem being heavily affected because their bodies do not match the image of a "perfect body." As Kenneth exclaimed:

> A perfect body is free of diseases! Although my body has not yet deteriorated I know that it is sick inside—full of virus. And who then is interested in me as a sexual being?

Others talk about their perception of losing their sexual attraction when symptoms start to develop. Robert who had lost a lot of weight said one day: "Look at my ass, it is *gone* and so is my sex appeal."

The necessity to carry a port-a-cath for medical reasons may also be a heavy blow to an individual's perception of being a sexual person. Many of the gay men said that the port-a-cath "takes away" their sexuality or in Philip's words: "Now when I've got that port-a-cath there is no question about it; that damn HIV robs me of everything including my sexual dignity." Robert expresses the situation in the following way:

> What do you think happens when the guy starts caressing my chest and realizes there is a bulk under the skin? Well, I know from experience that it will turn him off and most likely he just takes off.

Another man, Michael, got quite upset over some male pictures in our waiting room in Stockholm:

> It is very disturbing to me to look at these photos. These guys have such perfect bodies and there is no way for me to identify with them. Why don't they have at least a small

> KS lesion on their face or on their bodies? I feel ashamed about my body. My body isn't sexy. I feel like someone who the cat dragged into the house.

In other words, the "perfect body" attitude is by many men perceived as a mockery and threat to their self-image and self-esteem including sexual elements of self-esteem.

Bearing this in mind, it is not surprising that some gay men may undertake rigorous diets, exercises, and healthy living to develop a healthy, muscular body and in that way to pass as a healthy and sexual person. Exercise wards off illness but it also functions as a way to restore one's damaged self-image. In his book, Klitzman quotes a man, who captures that feeling in the following way:

> I feel victorious as a survivor going in to a bar and having everybody there want me.... I worked out, got in shape, cut my hair right, and learned how to look attractive. Now, they're all dying for me. One of my biggest dreams since I was 12 years old has been to have 20 more pounds of muscle, and I did it last year.[13] (p. 86–87)

Dementia or any brain lesions constitute a terrifying threat toward psychological survival. Robert indicates that: "I am terrified that the virus will attack my brain, because if it does that means that I would just vanish as a person." Simon told the therapist quite early on that he most feared developing brain lesions. One day when she visited him at the hospital, his eyes were sad, empty, and weary. He hardly spoke a word. The room shivered with his fear and horror. Eventually he told the therapist that he was to be given a CAT scan "to see what's going on in my brain. And as I have told you earlier I don't really recognize myself so this really scares the shit out of me." After these words Simon closed his eyes and shut off the external world.

To others, the great blow to their psychological survival would be to become dependent upon others. As Adam and Andy note respectively:

> I'd rather commit suicide than to become dependent upon others.

> To become really sick and to have to rely on others, no, that would be the same as losing my human dignity. I don't think I could cope with that.

Summary

The individual's physical survival is abruptly challenged by the HIV diagnosis and he is faced with a variety of physical threats. The clinical data showed that HIV-related concerns increased over time and that the meanings of the threats changed over the disease phases. In the asymptomatic phase the threats were time-related, whereas in the mild symptomatic phase the meaning was associated with bewilderment. The meaning turned into fear in the severe symptomatic phase and in the terminal phase into confirmation.

The HIV infection also threatens the individual's psychological survival because of the close link between the body and the self. Thus, the fear of losing one's self and self-esteem and ultimately dying psychologically is evoked.

SOCIAL THREATS

HIV infection is also a potential threat to the individual's social existence in terms of discrimination and aloneness, which are both manifestations of the stigmatization of HIV infection. The individual may suffer far more from the HIV stigma than the diagnosis in itself. Gay men with HIV are faced with 'multiple stigmatization,[15] that is, both in their role of being physically "sick" and as being gay. Social stigmatization is the result of anti-gay attitudes and the relationship between stigmatized gay behaviors and HIV. The "sickness" stigmatization originates from the associations between HIV, infectiousness, and death.

Weitz[16] argues that the social construction of HIV disease as a deserved punishment has led to discrimination, stigmatization, and rejection of people with HIV. The "deserved punishment" attitude is, as we see it, the result of the association between HIV and sexual desire, "promiscuity," loss of control, and forbidden eroticism, in particular the gay one. Such collective sexual dynamics call forth a combination of fascination and disgust but also a collective fear of loosing control over one's own unconscious sexual impulses.[17] These threatening impulses have to be warded off, and one way to do so is to project them into other people. People, who already have HIV, and in particular gay men, represent these sexual dynamics and become a good target for such projection.[18,19] The stronger the forbidden sexual impulses are the stronger prejudices toward, and detachment from, people with HIV become.

Discrimination and aloneness or "social death"[20] are among the negative consequences of disclosing one's HIV status.

Self-Disclosure

As HIV infection is a heavily stigmatized disease, self-disclosure is a charged issue for people living with HIV. As already stated in Chapter 3, self-disclosure refers to the individual's openness about his HIV status. Recent research reveals that disclosure is a potent stressor for many people with HIV, regardless of whether they choose to reveal their status.[21] But, as Holt et al. note, disclosure also acts as "a mechanism by which the individuals contend with their infection,"[21] (p. 58) and it may facilitate more effective coping and psychological adaptation to the disease. Disclosure is not a fixed state but rather a dynamic process.

In this section, we discuss self-disclosure as it relates to the social network domain, whereas the sexual domain is the focus of the following section.

People with HIV wrestle with when to tell as well as who to tell in their social network about their HIV status. The aim of the self-disclosure process is to come out about one's HIV seropositivity to significant others. Indirectly there is also a striving for interpersonal security and self-esteem,[22] self-acceptance, and regained control over one's life.[21] Some select carefully who to tell and still others feel they must "tell the world." The HIV-disclosure process may echo gay men's gay identity formation process,[23] in that the individual in both cases has to manage a stigmatized status. In Schwartzberg's words:

> being gay and being HIV positive may begin to interweave—in terms of how to manage self-disclosure, openness, pride, and shame; in terms of needing to once again acclimate to a world where the previous rules no longer apply.[24] (p. 36)

In the self-disclosure process the individual is confronted with the dilemma between, on the one hand, the psychological need for authenticity, affirmation, and respect, and on the other hand the fear of being rejected and abandoned when disclosing his HIV status, that is, to be "punished" when being authentic. Clinical and empirical data[21] indicate that in general self-disclosure is a result of a long and well thought-out process that takes into account contextual issues and appreciation of potential consequences of disclosure, both immediately and in the long term. Motives for disclosure within the social network may differ depending on who the potential "target" of disclosure is. Most often, the motive is to break the psychological isolation and/or a sense of denying and failing oneself. Another motive may be to live in accordance to the dictates of one's conscience or to stop rumors.

Holt et al.[21] observed in their study that whether or not to disclose one's HIV status was approached differently within the disease phases. At the early postdiagnostic phase the gay men adopted a policy of limited or nondisclosure. Such an approach provided the individual with time to "come to terms with" his diagnosis before having to contend with reactions from others. The asymptomatic person regarded disclosure as a matter of choice. Motives for disclosing were often a desire to regain control, to get appropriate social support, and to minimize stress related to nondisclosure. Those men who had developed symptoms or were diagnosed with AIDS were less reticent about disclosure, and they also employed disclosure to achieve self-acceptance through the acceptance of others. As with the asymptomatic men, those with symptoms or who were diagnosed with AIDS, disclosure within a sexual relationship was a means of sharing responsibility for "safer sex" as well as a marker of trust and intimacy. Further, data implied that only those men who had "come to accept their diagnosis" and had achieved self-acceptance were motivated to disclose their HIV seropositivity.

In some cases disclosing might not be carefully considered but rather be impulsive and be a reflection of internal psychological conflicts. One example of such a conflict would be to satisfy masochistic needs. Friedman has raised similar discussion in relation to coming out as gay.

> The sadistic aspects of homophobic society prove impossible for the masochistic person to resist. I am not suggesting that masochism provides a psychological model for coming out. I am pointing out, however, that gay masochistic patients, may use coming out in ways that have no real equivalent in heterosexual social-role behavior.[25] (p. 149)

But there are also individuals who decide not to disclose their HIV status to anyone. One contributing factor to being cautious about self-disclosure can be gay men's childhood and adolescence experiences of being rejected and deprived of affirmation. Fear of rejection, abandonment, disruption of social ties, and uncertainty over reactions of others are common sources for reluctance to tell others. Another source may be regret about bringing sadness to others, in particular parents and close friends. Others stress the private character of the matter. Some may socially withdraw for fear of "revealing" unintentionally their HIV status or as a consequence of a sense of HIV-related shame or lack of self-esteem.

By *not* sharing one's HIV status, feelings of having denied and failed oneself may appear and eventually lead to self-blame and reduced self-esteem. The individual is in a no-win situation. On the one hand, he needs support and on the other hand, he fears that seeking support will lead to rejection. Data show that the social network of gay men shrinks at the time of the HIV notification.[26–28] To some, this confirms that their fear of abandonment was "correct."

In the disclosing process one important element may be to seek out others in the same situation or in self-psychological terminology to seek twinship bonds (i.e., the experience of feeling an essential alikeness with others).[29] Some gay men become active within body positive groups/organizations supplying them with a feeling of subculture and belonging. Positive reinforcement and the social and psychological support of others provide confidence and may facilitate disclosure. Another facilitator may be the psychotherapeutic context. Harald is an example of this.

Harald was a man in his mid-forties who had been married and had children. He came out as gay about ten years prior to his HIV diagnosis but expressed strong internalized antihomosexual attitudes (i.e., internalized homophobia). When Harald initiated the therapeutic contact, he had known about his HIV seropositivity for one year. He was an insecure person and afraid to assert himself in different situations, including his workplace. His self-image was negative. During the first year, the focus of the therapeutic work was very much on these issues, and slowly Harald started to become more assertive and to view himself in less negative terms. In parallel to his self-development, which was an ongoing theme over the years, Harald also struggled with self-disclosure. He started to develop severe symptoms and was diagnosed with AIDS in the course of the second year. At the same time, he started to consider whether he should disclose his HIV status to someone within his family of origin. He told one of his siblings and was well received. During the following semester, Harald was quite occupied with existential concerns and the sense of being under pressure from the "AIDS stone." He decided to tell his ex-wife about his HIV condition and received the same positive support as with his sibling. More and more, Harald was on sick leave and he therefore decided to disclose his AIDS diagnosis to his supervisor. The response was to make re-arrangements in Harald's work tasks. Harald reacted strongly, and after a few weeks, he decided to speak up at his workplace and eventually he was able to return to his original tasks. The third year was very much characterized by the roller-coaster phenomenon. Toward the end of the third year, Harald experienced the feeling that he was in control of his HIV and felt responsible for his life. Within this context he told his children about his HIV and got very strong support.

What does the clinical scene look like with respect to self-disclosure? Among the Swedish gay men, it was an infrequently mentioned topic, although about 50% of the men at some time discussed the issues. Those men who brought it up were in the asymptomatic or mild symptomatic phase and their concerns were mostly related to when and in what ways to disclose their HIV status to their parents and/or colleagues. This finding might seem odd given what has been stated earlier about people wrestling with this question. One explanation could be that all except four of the men had learned about their HIV serostatus at least two years (time range of one to nine years) prior to the therapeutic contact and might thus at least to some extent have already dealt with this issue. The figures might have been quite different if the initial contact had taken place closer in time to learning about their HIV seropositivity.

Discrimination

There is no doubt that self-disclosure can have negative consequences, such as discrimination in the workplace, in health care systems, and insurance matters. In Sweden, at the time of writing—in contrast to the United States—HIV infection does not qualify for the protection of the antidiscrimination law.* But the Swedish protective employment law states that disease is not a legal cause of notice of termination provided the person has tenure. Reality shows, however, that legislation does not necessarily protect people from discrimination. Employers in the United States, for example, appear to feel free to neglect workers' rights to nondiscrimination and fire employees because of their HIV infection. Discrimination may also take place in more subtle, indirect ways and therefore be much more difficult to demonstrate. Negative remarks about people with HIV or AIDS, jokes, and patronizing, demeaning attitudes are other examples of "informal" discrimination.

Another discriminatory attitude occurs when people with HIV are transferred at work from one post to another out of "consideration" or "the best-for-you" attitude. Among the men with whom Dr. Schönnesson has worked psychotherapeutically over the years, discrimination in work settings as a result of self-disclosure is rare.

Discrimination may also appear when it comes to participation in various alternative psychological therapies. Michael disclosed his HIV status when applying to a weekend course. However, he was informed that he was not welcome

*HIV is classified as a disability in Sweden, and as of May 1, 1999, those with disabilities are protected from discrimination in Sweden.

because there would be "a lot of sweat and tears" and the leader considered Michael as being a risk to others in the group!

Discrimination, like self-disclosure, was an infrequently mentioned topic, although more than two-thirds of the men at some time brought it up.

It has to be remembered though, that responses to self-disclosure can also be supportive and caring. Under such conditions, common remarks are: "It is like a great big relief"; "Why didn't I do it earlier?"; "It's like tons of bricks off my shoulders"; and "I feel empowered."

Aloneness

The fear of aloneness or interpersonal isolation[30] lurks not only in the self-disclosure decision process but also after disclosure. The fear is understandable considering the importance of relationships for human beings' psychological survival and well-being. Bowlby writes:

> Intimate attachments to other human beings are the hub around which a person's life evolves, not only when he is an infant or a toddler or a schoolchild but throughout his adolescence and his years of maturity as well, and on into old age. From these intimate attachments a person draws his strength and enjoyment of life and, through what he contributes, he gives strength and enjoyment to others. These are matters about which current science and traditional wisdom are at one.[31] (p. 442)

From a self-psychological perspective[29] relationships are crucial in establishing the individual's self. In the development of the self there is a constant separation from certain relations and a constant seeking of other relations. Each relationship has a function in terms of meeting the individual's mirroring, twinship, and idealizing needs (referred to as selfobject functions in the psychoanalytic literature). Mirroring refers to our need for affirmation and recognition from others. Twinship needs contain the experience of feeling an essential alikeness with others. Finally, idealizing describes the experience of being soothed, protected, and accepted by an admired and respected person but also by ideas and symbols. Philosopher Martin Buber[32] argues along the same lines in proclaiming that "in the beginning is the relation" and that "there is no 'I' as such, but only the basic word 'I—Thou'." We also have to bear in mind that an anti-gay society complicates gay men's self-development, a topic we address in Chapter 9.

We want to emphasize though that the fear and experiences of interpersonal isolation may be reinforced, colored, and compounded by earlier psychological conflicts and problems. Sometimes the individual "blames" HIV for his intimacy problems, although with closer examination these problems have existed long before the HIV diagnosis. Eric suffered a lot from not having a steady partner. He argued that it was a consequence of his HIV status "no one wants me because I'm HIV positive." He decided to socially withdraw because "I have given up the idea of finding someone." In due course he realized that adult intimacy had always been a problem to him, but "it was so much easier to blame HIV for that than to scrutinize myself."

Two-thirds of the gay men experienced aloneness. These experiences were more or less salient over all four phases of the disease (the asymptomatic, the mild symptomatic, the severe symptomatic, and the terminal phase). The men talked about aloneness in terms of being abandoned and a sense of being invisible. The latter emotion has an existential quality in that it represents a sense of being no one, that is, to experience psychological death, as discussed in Chapter 7. Those men, who were in the final disease phase, tended also to be occupied with thoughts about being an outsider. From a physical perspective, the advanced disease process may severely limit social interaction and the sick person may express fear of becoming completely socially isolated. Norman was very afraid that his friends would not like to be around him "because I really look like death."

Gay men with HIV may also display worries that their homosocial existence is threatened. As one respondent in Ross and Ryan's study indicated:

> And I've had a couple of bad experiences whereby you open up ... you tell someone, trying to be honest, that you're HIV and the reaction is quite extraordinary, and someone said to me the other day that the most anti-HIV people is in the (gay) community.[20] (p. 14)

Another way to put it is the experience of an "us" and "them" subculture. Hubert indicates:

> I would say that the community is divided into "us," that's us with HIV and "them" referring to those who are assumed to be HIV negative. I often feel like a third-class gay in gay bars and I'm often looked upon as an outcast. Sometimes I get the feeling that people who are HIV negative don't think that we who are HIV positive mingle with the HIV negative community, No, we should be in the hospital or we are so depressed that we are at home. A complete separation between the worlds in other words.

Jeffrey, a 40-year-old gay man, long-term nonprogressor, expresses a variation on the two worlds:

> It is amazing to realize that because I have a beer belly, wear a suit, tie, and carry a briefcase, many potential partners don't believe me when I tell them I am HIV positive. Their response is that "you can't be that, you look so healthy."

As a response to these worries of exclusion from or peripheral status in gay subcultures, gay men with HIV may decide to only socialize with other men they know have HIV. As Roger points out:

> I prefer to spend my time with other people who are positive. They know what I am going through, they understand me without me having to explain everything.

Multiple Loss

Another potential threat to social existence is the multiple loss and accompanying grief that so many gay men experience. Cho and Cassidy, as quoted by

Maasen,[33] define multiple loss as "chronic bereavement that involves not only chronic grief, but also anticipatory grief and unresolved grief, and the experience of several losses simultaneously." It is not unusual to hear men saying that they lost more than 50 friends and acquaintances over the years. There is no equivalent to such an experience in the nongay subcultures (except possibly in wartime or disasters). HIV and AIDS represent in the gay communities an irreparable, incomprehensible loss. Jacoby Klein[34] stresses that the multiple loss is magnified in gay subcultures, as they tend to be "closed systems," which are a consequence of societal antihomosexual attitudes (i.e., societal homophobia). On a communal level the losses are related to the loss of gay cultural norms and styles of sexual expression. "AIDS has infused the sorrow of old age into individuals and communities"[24] (p. 66). As Robert Gluck puts it (cited in Weeks):

> AIDS creates such magnitude of *loss* that now death is where gay men experience life most keenly as a group. It's where we learn about love, where we discover new values and qualities in ourselves. Death joins if not replaces sex as the community sublime.[7] (p. 45)

On the personal level the losses are associated to the deaths of beloved and liked people and consequently the individual's social network deteriorates. As Robert said during a session:

> All my friends are dead and it feels like I have no roots any more. There is no one there for me, no one to share my history with. And I don't have the energy to get to know new men who are HIV positive. Besides most of them are newly diagnosed, so when I talk about the 1980s they just look at me like an alien.

Repeated grief experiences contribute to worries of committing oneself to new relationships out of fear of being abandoned again, which may induce social withdrawal. As Charles states: "I can't stand another death so I prefer to be on my own or at least try to avoid getting involved in someone on a deeper level." Thus social isolation of choice can function as a protective shelter toward anticipated separation and emotional suffering. Others may be in conflict as they express their feelings of isolation and abandonment while they simultaneously withdraw from social support networks.

Summary

The HIV infection is also a potential threat to the individual's social existence in terms of discrimination, aloneness, and multiple loss. Both discrimination and aloneness are potential negative consequences of openness about HIV status and are manifestations of the stigma attached to HIV. Discrimination is of a formal as well as an informal character and aloneness usually relates to being abandoned and a sense of being invisible. Self-disclosure as well as discrimination was mentioned, although infrequently, by most of the gay men in the clinical setting. Feelings of aloneness appeared to be more or less salient in all four disease phases. Dr.

Schönnesson's data also indicate that many gay men worried about being excluded or getting a peripheral status in any of the gay subcultures. Finally, experiences of multiple loss of friends and acquaintances threaten the social network with deterioration.

SEXUAL THREATS

Foucault[35] argues that sex has become "the truth of our being," the core of an essential self. A similar view is held by Weeks[7] who emphasizes that the sexual has been a prime site for the struggle for a sense of self and identity. This perspective is reflected in the gay satellite culture in which sexuality is central and thus pivotal to quality of life as well. To some gay men sexuality is an important base of their identity and self-esteem.[20] Nicholas, for example, feels totally rejected as a human being when his sexual partners do not want to kiss (french kissing) him. The individual sexuality has different gestalts (or representations). It is a site of danger and pleasure and as a response to HIV its gay identification gestalt has changed into one of great potential danger and anxiety.

In times when the individual's psychological equilibrium is threatened, he needs a shield that serves to restabilize the equilibrium. The individual's sexuality can, as a compensation strategy, play an important role in this process. Schorsch[36] speaks about two compensatory aspects: the narcissistic and the psychological reproductive aspects. The narcissistic aspect refers to the role of sex as a psychological stabilizer (or a distracting mechanism) by, for example, smothering depression and anxiety, reducing tension, and increasing (but also masking low) self-esteem. This aspect appears to be quite familiar to many of the gay men in the clinical study. Some of the men talked about their need to have sex in order to "fill my sense of emptiness." Others reflected over their past (pre-HIV) sexual encounters, such as Peter:

> I've started to think about why I had so much sex. Because now I can see that I didn't want to have that much sex. But it was, I think, a way for me to get close to someone. I wanted something else, I can see that now, I wanted intimacy, but I didn't know then how to get that except through having as much sex as possible. I certainly fooled myself.

The psychological reproductive aspect alludes to irrational fantasies about "life reproduction." Sexuality receives a symbolic existential value, as counterweight to death, symbolizing life and its continuity. To be sexual is associated with hope of a future and a longing to avoid death.

The salience of concerns related to potential "sexual death"[20] is illuminated in that all but five of the 38 men talked frequently about their sexual concerns, regardless of disease phase. The individual's sexual existence, in terms of sexual behaviors, intimacy, and gay identity and lifestyle, is in the course of the infection exposed to HIV-related psychological, social, and medical threats.

Sexual Behaviors

Persons with HIV are faced with two major sexual dilemmas that bear significance on their sexual existence. One is related to protected sex and the other to self-disclosure of one's HIV status. These dilemmas may be compounded by a sense of being plague-stricken, nonattractive, and not "good enough" as a sexual individual and by society's denial of their sexuality. In addition, HIV disease progression and physical deterioration may have an impact on sexual desire, physical functioning, and sexual ability.

The Protected Sex Dilemma

The core of the HIV sexual behavioral scenario is to find a psychological equilibrium between protected sex and sexual well-being. This is a continuing process and to many the equilibrium has to be recaptured over and over again. There are demands and expectations on people with HIV to change their sexual riskful behaviors into less risky ones (i.e., to practice protected sex) and to maintain these changes throughout the rest of their lives. These expectations are a potential source of stress and frustration. As Thomas comments: "You know, I carry this heavy burden of *never* being allowed to loose control or to make any mistakes. I am simply not allowed to be human."

Even when protected sex is practiced there is a degree of uncertainty or anxiety in terms of condom failure or concerns about transmission of HIV through oral sex. Gerald emphasized at a point in his therapy: "Do you realize that I am a potential murderer even though I practice safer sex?!"

Within the public health policy context persons with HIV are also held responsible for always practicing protected sex (in the case of unknown or negative status of the partner). However, some men, as illustrated by Rex, complain about the "one-way person" responsibility. Rex is amazed that:

> so few of the guys out there talk and even less so initiate using condoms. It's like they think that people with HIV don't have sex. They just don't seem to care. So if I don't use the condom, well, there would be unsafe sex. I find it so hard sometimes to always be the one to take the responsibility.

Therefore, some decide to withdraw sexually, at least temporarily.

The sexual behavioral dilemma of gay men with HIV is very often looked upon from solely a cognitive and rational perspective. In order to do justice to the complexity of sexual behavior change, we also have to address the psychological aspects of the individual's sexuality. First, we must be aware that people create sexual behavioral scripts that may differ from situation to situation and from partner to partner. Some of the behaviors are perceived as more pleasurable than others and some are more important than others to sexual satisfaction.[37] Consequently, to change one's sexual life pattern that lends joy, pleasure, and satisfaction is not easy. It is surprising that so little research has been done on the sexual pleasure/importance dimensions of sexuality. Those few studies that do exist show that when unprotected sex is related to sexual pleasure or sexual importance, it is more difficult to refrain from.[37–39]

Another important psychological aspect is the boundless or regressive dimension of sexuality; that is, to give in physically and psychologically to another person without any constraints. A person living with HIV is, due to the infectiousness of HIV, debarred from this dimension. In other words, psychological suffering within the sexual context is not only related to reduced hedonism because of behavioral changes and/or behavioral giving up, it also relates to the individual's awareness that sexual boundlessness has to be replaced by sexual boundary. There seems to be a paradox here. It was argued earlier that the sexual act gets an existential value in that it symbolizes life and its continuity, that is, it is a counterweight for death. But when the individual practices protected sex the sexual act symbolizes death in its boundary function.

A third psychological aspect is the psychological representations of sexual behaviors. Unprotected anal sex represents to many gay men (regardless of HIV status) intimacy, a merger with one's partner, and trust, and therefore, condoms are perceived as a barrier to intimacy.

Bearing in mind that protected sex implies relinquished hedonistic, boundless, and symbolic meaning of one's sexuality, it is then understandable that sexual behavioral changes are to most people linked with feelings of loss, suffering, rage, grief and its accompanying mourning. To those gay men whose identification is strongly vested in sexual performance, sexual behavioral changes may be construed as an "identity death."[20] It is notable that our empirical knowledge is almost nonexistent with respect to what extent gay men with HIV may experience psychological and/or sexual distress as a consequence of their sexual behavior changes.

The Self-Disclosure Dilemma

Another potential source of stress and frustration is the public health policy and ethical issues in relation to self-disclosure. In Sweden, this policy is legalized in the Communicable Disease Act as HIV is classified as a venereal and a reportable disease to infectious disease officers. The law requires disclosure of one's HIV seropositivity as well as condom use when practicing anal, oral, or vaginal intercourse. If the consulting physician has reason to suppose that a patient does not comply or will not comply with these instructions, he must promptly notify the county medical officer. The latter should try to obtain voluntary compliance from the patient before resorting to coercive measures. If these actions are not followed, despite repeated summons, the county medical officer can appeal to the county administrative court, which may decide on an order for compulsory isolation. Compulsory isolation may continue for up to three months but can exceed that time limit.

Many Swedish gay men with HIV perceive the legal information duty in combination with the threat of potential custody as a stressor and an obstacle to sexual well-being. There is also the fear that a sexual partner might report the man with HIV for having had unprotected sex—even though that might not be true. "The guy might be pissed off with me for some reasons so this is an excellent way to take revenge on me."

The core of the self-disclosure dilemma is (like disclosure to social networks) fear of rejection and social isolation. To be rejected as a sexual person is a hard blow for one's self and self-esteem and may lead to feelings of being a no one, particularly if one's central identity is "being a gay man." The individual is faced with the difficult decision of the timing of disclosure in the sexual context in order to run the lowest risk of being rejected. This is highlighted in the following reflection from Paul:

> Is there actually any critical timing when one would run the lowest risk to be rejected? When are the partner or I mature enough for disclosure? I think this is very difficult because it is so unpredictable how the other will react upon it. It is always a hell of a struggle.

Some men are afraid that if they disclose their HIV seropositivity to their sexual partner he may spread the information to others and "then I am doomed when it comes to new sexual partners." Peter expresses his suspicion toward the gay subcultures in general: "HIV is still kind of a big thing and you know there are plenty of bitches out there. Nothing would stop them from gossiping about my status."

"Solutions" of the Sexual Dilemmas

The sexual dilemmas can be "solved" in different ways. The solutions are not necessarily fixed but may change over time contingent upon intrapersonal factors and social/sexual contexts. With respect to disclosure the individual may decide not to tell anyone or to always inform the sexual partners. Others decide not to inform casual partners as long as protected sex is practiced, whereas potential steady partners are always told. The protected sex dilemma may be "solved" by means of continuing with unprotected sex. Another solution is to make the behavioral changes and to practice sexual behaviors that are negatively loaded. Still another way is to change the sexual risky practices and to find new, nonrisky positively loaded ways of expressing one's sexual desire.

Sexual abstinence or self-quarantine is another solution. Within Dr. Schönnesson's clinical practice, some men have withdrawn sexually because the sexual behavioral changes and/or self-disclosure carry too high of a psychological price. Kenneth argues: "To have sex? No, it's simply not worth it—all the hazards and the concerns and worries." Self-quarantine may also be generated by fear of rejection, abandonment, perception of blame and guilt, and discredited identity.

To others the "next to the optimal" solution is to restrict one's cruising areas to the Body Positive group, a volunteer organization of gay and bisexual men living with HIV.

Medical Threats

Clinical experiences and empirical studies (albeit still rare) show that HIV infection may have a negative impact on sexual desire, organic functioning, or ability. Research findings[12,40,41] indicate that a decreased interest and desire and difficulties in both maintaining an erection and in achieving ejaculation were reported by one-third of gay men with HIV and two-thirds of gay men with AIDS. Another study[42] found that those gay men living with HIV, more often than their HIV seronegative counterparts, reported a decline in sexual interest and sexual pleasure and erectile difficulties.

Another poorly explored research area is to what extent HIV-related physiological treatment, medical treatment, and/or psychosocial factors contribute to decreased sexual interest, sexual desire, impaired sexual functioning, and/or sexual disability. In Meyer-Bahlburg et al.'s study[42] none of the sexual symptoms were related to HIV disease phases. Tindall et al., on the other hand, argue that given the fact that "the majority of reported dysfunction occurred both during masturbation and with sexual partners" it suggests that it is "primarily related to organic rather than situational or psychogenic factors."[41] (p. 106)

Intimacy

As stated earlier in this chapter, there is a strong emphasis on intimate relationship in our Western culture. Among those 38 gay men whose psychotherapeutic notes were analyzed, 12 of them never engaged in a love relationship over the time they were in therapy. Some of them expressed a strong yearning for one, though they found the infection such an insurmountable barrier that love relationships were perceived as unattainable to them. The barrier was not necessarily the infection in itself (i.e., the fear of transmission), but the barrier was associated with its negative psychological and social consequences, such as a negative self-image reflected in the following quote: "I'm a minority within a minority and no one wants me." To others the barrier was equal to the individual's sense of not being worthy to be loved or to love. Still others were so afraid to disclose their HIV status that they in no way dared to expose themselves to potential partners. Usually there was a combination of different barrier representations involved in the decision. In other words these men's intimate dimension is indeed threatened by HIV.

It has been estimated that between 30% and 60% of gay men are in primary committed relationships.[43] It has to be stressed though that gay couples, in contrast to straight couples, are exposed to specific stressors related to their same gender preference. They may experience negative attitudes and be looked upon as "deviant," and lack support, validation, and acknowledgment of their needs within the relationship. In those male couples where one or both members have HIV, the intensity of this experience is magnified.[44] Although we are aware that HIV infection has introduced a tragic element into the lives of many gay couples, distressingly little attention has been paid to psychosocial and psychosexual consequences of and strains on the relationship. The sparsely existing empirical research has focused on gay couples of serodiscordant HIV status.[45] It is fairly safe to assume that this "population" is of greater concern to public health interest because of the potential risk of HIV transmission. We think this attitude is unfortunate in that gay couples with HIV-seropositive concordance status run the risk of being excluded from psychological and health care concerns. These couples struggle with the same external and relational issues and stressors that their discordant counterpart does. This is clearly demonstrated in the quantitative analysis of the psychotherapeutic notes. Of those 26 men who in the course of the therapeutic contact were engaged in a love relationship, eight men were in a serodiscordant status relationship whereas the others were involved in HIV-seroconcordant relationships. All but one of them brought up and talked frequently about relational issues. It is notable that these issues declined (but not significantly) in their salience in the severe symptomatic phase (phase 3) and the final phase (phase 4) of the disease. This finding is not a manifestation of separation from the partner, but we argue a reflection of having worked through many of the relational issues.

Empirical data and our own clinical experiences indicate that relational issues such as communication, conflicts, and commitment that typically confront any couple are usually exacerbated in couples with HIV. In addition the couple is faced with specific HIV-related stressors linked not only to the disease domain but also to the sexual and social domains of the relationship. Powell-Cope argues that being part of a couple affected by HIV is perceived as:

> a major life transition as both partners are confronted with multiple losses including the possible death of the person with AIDS, dissolution of the relationship, health, independence, intimacy, and privacy.[46] (p. 36)

The Disease Domain

HIV infection has been, and still is, to many associated with uncertainty, shortened life expectancy, and death. Protease inhibitors and combination therapies have not taken away uncertainty, but its gestalt has changed. Earlier uncertainty was very much linked to a matter of time of death and continued life was not an option. Today uncertainty appears to be associated with whether life will conquer death or vice versa. But uncertainty is also related to what future patterns of HIV-related symptoms and diseases will look like. Medications, their side effects, and potential consequences for health are also a source of uncertainty. In those couples where both men have HIV it is quite common to hear them expressing uncertainty with respect to who is to "take care of me, to console me when my partner is dead."

Closely linked to uncertainty are difficulties related to future planning in terms of career, savings, housing, travel, and so forth. The perception that one is restricted in long-term planning, in contrast to couples not living with HIV, is experienced as a significant loss. It can evoke anger, despair, and feelings of injustice—"it is not fair that we have to live with this uncertainty." It is not uncommon that couples express feelings of hopelessness about their future as a couple, that their relationship will not last until old age.

Regardless of the HIV status of the couple there is an imbalance (more pronounced in serodisconcordant status) as to life expectancy between the two partners. Within the couple of serodisconcordant status, it may invoke envy within the person with HIV—"It drives me nuts knowing that he will survive me." The person who is HIV negative may on his behalf experience a sense of survival guilt. When both men have HIV sometimes a reciprocal psychological "competition" for who is the sicker can be observed. One man in Dr. Schönnesson's clinical practice, Arthur, was very distressed over his partner who "always" regarded himself as the sicker of the two and expected Arthur to always be there for him. Arthur had a strong sense that his partner used his disease as a tool for blackmail. Other couples have more or less outspoken discussions about who would be the one to die first. Bob and Charles had lived together for many years. Bob was an outgoing person, whereas Charles was more introverted. Bob often argued that it would be much better if Charles died before him because "Charles doesn't have that many friends as I have and I would cope with his death much better than he would with mine." Bob died first.

Dying and death are other topics that are heavily charged. The clinical impression is that the couples rarely talk about the final total separation. But there are exceptions. Nicholas and William had constantly avoided the topic up until exactly (to the day) two months prior to Nicholas's death. At that moment, they spelled out their fears of Nicholas's impending death and they summarized their long-term love relationship. Nicholas and William were in agreement that William would care for Nicholas in their home where Nicholas also wanted to die.

Another potential stressor within the disease domain is caretaking concerns.[47,48] The partner has in his caretaker role a dual responsibility as a primary partner as well as a "nurse." It is a well-known fact from studying other diseases that this combination is usually very taxing on a relationship. One aspect of caretaking is the sick person's development of dependency in the course of progression, which may trigger emotions such as anger, despair, hopelessness, guilt, and vulnerability. The caregiver may feel that he is "trapped" and may experience guilt feelings when he prioritizes himself.

The Social Domain

One aspect of the social domain is openness about the couple's HIV status. When the couple is not "out" to family, friends, and colleagues or disagrees about whether and if so when to tell others, it is a stressor on the relationship.[49] It can happen in couples with serodisconcordant serostatus that the noninfected man, without his partner's consent, tells some of his own friends or someone within their joint circle of friends about his partner's HIV seropositivity. The burden of being the only one to know about the partner's serostatus is exemplified in the following. Hubert complained:

> I can't carry it all alone on my shoulders. It's just too much. I need someone to turn to, someone outside our relationship with whom I can talk to about the situation.

One reaction from the person with HIV to the partner's disclosure is a sense of betrayal. Andrew reacted in quite another way. He told his partner, James, that he did not "like it and I can't change it. Done is done." Andrew's response was to never again meet the informed friend. The rationale behind the decision was that Andrew was absolutely convinced that the friend would completely change his attitude toward him and take on a "pity and no respect-attitude," which Andrew "could not stand."

The danger of secrecy of HIV is that the couple becomes socially isolated.[50] On the other hand, couples (like the individual) also run the risk of being rejected and experiencing lack of support and validation of their relationship when families and/or friends are informed about their HIV status. Still the couples who participated in Mattison and McWhirter's study[49] emphasized the importance of reaching out to friends but also to mobilizing a professional social supportive network. Other couples are confronted with illness and death of their gay friends and experience bereavement processes. As Mattison and McWhirter point out, "each instance of illness and death of friends or acquaintances forces the couple to confront the prospects of death"[49] (p. 94).

The Sexual Domain

A potential stressor within couples with serodisconcordant status is the need to always practice protected sex to avoid HIV transmission. However, both clinical experiences and empirical data[49,51–54] show that some couples do not adhere to these guidelines. Others use condoms inconsistently during the course of a single sexual activity and still others have periodic unprotected sex within a steady relationship. Within the protected sex context, we should be aware of the paradox of condom use,[55] that is, the condom is a protection from HIV transmission and at the same time it is a reminder of the risk of HIV. The main reasons for not adhering to protected sex appear to be related to intimacy aspects. It is common among gay men that the condom is perceived as a barrier to intimacy. Unprotected sex may symbolize commitment and investment in the relationship,[56] a desire for the noninfected partner to "join my lover in being in this thing together," a belief that "true love will conquer all," "accidents of passion," alcohol, or drugs.

There are also other potential sexual stressors within couples. Within some couples (regardless of their HIV status) there is disagreement with respect to practicing unprotected/protected sex. There are also noninfected members who are too afraid of HIV transmission to practice even protected sex and/or other non-penetrative sexual activities. This situation may evoke within the partner with HIV feelings of being dangerous, nonattractive, not loved, and so forth. As stated before the sexual domain may also be threatened by medical conditions, which may have an impact on sexual desire, functioning, and ability.

Summary

The above-discussed stressors within the disease, social, and sexual domains are in themselves a strain to the couple. In addition it is quite common for the members of the couple to perceive these stressors diversely as to their heaviness, complexity, and salience but also in timing, which may lead to further conflicts within the relationship. It is, however, our impression, which is supported by empirical findings,[48,50] that talking about HIV and its related topics is often avoided in both serodiscordant and HIV seropositive concordant couples. Re-occurring reasons for not discussing these topics are disclaimers of not wanting to worry or upset the other or hurt or make him feel bad or put a burden on the other. Instead of talking the couple withdraws into silence and frustration with all their emotions to protect each other from HIV-related concerns and/or fantasies. Paradoxically, this avoidant attitude may aggravate conflicts and difficulties within the relationship. But we have to acknowledge that at the bottom line of the avoidant attitude is the fear of rejection and ultimately separation.

Gay Identity and Lifestyle

The sexual culture of the gay person has co-existed with, and to some degree defined, the identity of the gay.[20] But the gay is also the homosocial. However, the sexual and the social circles are interwoven as gay interaction often takes place in specific gay venues. The merger of the two arenas may have a negative impact on gay men with HIV and their participation/commitment/investment in the gay subcultures. For example when the man perceives himself less attractive he is less inclined to be part of the social scene and by withdrawing from it he also withdraws from the sexual scene. The individual may also withdraw from gay friends because of depression, low self-esteem, fear of being abandoned, or guilt and shame. This may lead to loss of subcultural support. An additional scenario is when the gay man's friends reject him due to his HIV status.

Another situation is when confrontation with cumulative losses is so burdensome that it may trigger negative evaluations of a gay lifestyle.[57,58] As Norman expressed during a session: "I'm sick and tired of the gay scene. It is only surrounded by disease and death and I'm looking for healthy people." Gay men who withdraw from gay subcultures run the risk of loosing homosocial contact, interaction, and support and in that way experience social death.[20]

Summary

The individual's sexual existence in terms of sexual behaviors, intimacy, and gay identity and lifestyle is exposed to HIV-related psychological, social, and medical threats. With respect to sexual behaviors, the person with HIV is faced with two major sexual dilemmas. One is related to protected sex and the other to self-disclosure of one's HIV status. In addition, HIV disease progression and physical deterioration may have an impact on sexual desire, physical functioning, and sexual ability.

The intimacy dimension may also be threatened. Psychological and social HIV-related concerns may pose insurmountable barriers to initiate and engage in love relationships. For those men who were in a love relationship, relational issues such as communication, conflicts, and commitment were usually exacerbated. In addition, the couple was faced with specific HIV-related stressors linked to the disease, sexual, and social domains of the relationship.

The gay identity and lifestyle are also exposed to HIV-related stressors. As the sexual and the social circles are interwoven in the gay scene, it may have a negative impact on gay men with HIV and their participation in the gay subcultures. When the man perceives himself as less attractive and/or less well-off psychologically, he is less inclined to be part of the social scene and thus he also withdraws from the sexual scene. His withdrawal may lead to loss of subcultural support.

REFERENCES

1. Hacking I. *Rewriting the Soul. Multiple Personality and the Sciences of Memory*. Princeton, N.J.: Princeton University Press; 1995.
2. Lazarus RS, Folkman S. *Stress, Appraisal, and Coping*. New York: Springer; 1984.
3. Janoff-Bulman R. *Shattered assumptions. Towards a New Psychology of Trauma*. New York: Free Press; 1995.
4. *Diagnostic and Statistical Manual of Mental Disorders, DSM IV*. Washington D.C.: American Psychiatric Association; 1994.
5. Lifton RJ. The concept of the survivor. In: Dimsdale JF, ed. *Survivors, Victims, and Perpetrators: Essays on the Nazi Holocaust*. Washington D.C.: Hemisphere; 1980.
6. Hammelstein P. How gay men cope with HIV infection—A review of German literature. *ALGP Europé Newsletter* 1996; 5(2):7–9.

7. Weeks, J. *Invented Moralities. Sexual Values in an Age of Uncertainty.* New York: Columbia University Press; 1996.
8. Rabkin J, Remien RH, Wilson C. *Good Doctors Good Patients. Partners in HIV Treatment.* New York: NCM Publishers; 1994.
9. Maasen T. Lacking the lust for extended gay life: counselling gay survivors of the AIDS epidemic from a psychodynamic view. Paper presented at the 2nd European conference on the methods and results of social and behavioral research on AIDS, Paris January 12–15, 1998.
10. Winiarski MG, ed. *HIV Mental Health for the 21st Century.* New York: New York University Press; 1997.
11. Klein SJ. *Heavenly Hurts. Surviving AIDS-Related Deaths and Losses.* Death, Value, and Meaning series. New York: Baywood Publishing; 1997.
12. Nilsson Schönnesson L. HIV infection: Trauma, psychic metabolism, and psychological well-being. A study of 29 Swedish gay HIV-positive men. Unpublished research report (in Swedish). Stockholm; 1993
13. Klitzman, R. *Being Positive: The Lives of Men and Women with HIV.* Chicago: Ivan R. Dee; 1997.
14. Kierkegaard S. *The Concept of Dread.* Princeton, N.J.: Princeton University Press; 1944.
15. Goffman E. *Stigma. Notes on the Management of Spoiled Identity.* Englewood Cliffs, N.J.: Prentice-Hall; 1963.
16. Weitz R. *Life with AIDS.* New Brunswick, N.J.: Rutgers University Press; 1992.
17. Schmidt G. Moral und Volksgesundheit. In: Sigusch V, ed. *Aids als Risiko.* Hamburg: Kronkret Literatur Verlag; 1987; 24–38.
18. Stevens LA, Muskin PR. Techniques for reversing failure of empathy towards AIDS patients. *Journal of the American Academy of Psychoanalysis* 1987; 15:539–551.
19. Becker S. AIDS—die Krankheit zur Wende? *Psychologie Heute* 1985; 12:60–65.
20. Ross MW, Ryan L. The little deaths: perceptions of HIV, sexuality, and quality of life in gay men. In: Ross MW, ed. *HIV/AIDS and Sexuality.* New York: Harrington Park Press; 1995; 1–21.
21. Holt R, Court P, Vedhara K, *et al.* The role of disclosure in coping with HIV infection. *AIDS Care* 1998; 10(1):49–60.
22. Sullivan HS. *Personal Psychopathology.* New York: Norton; 1972.
23. Ross MW, Tebble WEM, Viliunas D. Staging of psychological reactions to HIV infection in asymptomatic gay men. *Journal of Psychology and Human Sexuality* 1989; 2(1):93–104.
24. Schwartzberg S. *A Crisis of Meaning. How Gay Men Are Making Sense of AIDS.* New York: Oxford University Press; 1996.
25. Friedman RC. *Male Homosexuality. A Contemporry Psychoanalytic Perspective.* New Haven and London: Yale University Press; 1988.
26. Schaefer A, Paar G, Siedenbiedel W, *et al.* Psychosocial correlates of a four-month group therapy in HIV-positives, gay and bisexual men. Presented at the IXth international Conference on AIDS, June, Berlin; 1993.
27. Kaisch K, Anton-Culver H. Psychological and social consequences of HIV exposure: Gays in Southern California. *Psychology and Health* 1989; 3:63–75.
28. Wolcott D, Namir S, Fawzy, FI, *et al.* Illness concerns, attitudes towards homosexuality, and social support in gay men with AIDS. *General Hospital Psychiatry* 1986; 8:395–403.
29. Kohut H. *The Analysis of the Self.* New York: International Universities Press; 1971.
30. Yalom I. *Existential Psychotherapy.* New York: Basic Books; 1980.
31. Bowlby J. *Loss, Sadness and Depression: Attachment and Loss.* Vol. 3. New York: Basic Books; 1980.
32. Buber M. *I and Thou.* New York: Charles Schribner; 1970.
33. Maasen, T. Counseling gay men with multiple loss and survival problems: the breavement group as a transitional object. *AIDS Care* 1998; 10(1):S57–S63.
34. Jacoby Klein, S. AIDS-related multiple loss syndrome. *Illness, Crisis and Loss* 1994; 4(1):13–25.

35. Foucault M. *The History of Sexuality*, Vol. 1, *An Introduction*. London: Allen Lane; 1979.
36. Schorsch V. Die Theorie der Liebe in der Sexualwissenschaft. In *Sexualität: Vorträge im Wintersemester 1986/87*. Ruprecht-Karls Univesität: Heidelberg: Studium Generale; 1989.
37. Nilsson Schönnesson L, Dolezal C. HIV-related risk factors among Swedish gay men. *Scandinavian Journal of Sexology* 1998; 1:1:51–62.
38. Ekstrand MI, Coates TJ. Maintenance of safer sexual behaviors and predictors of risky-sex The San Francisco men's health study. *American Journal of Public Health* 1990; 80:973–977.
39. Stall RD, Ekstrand MI, Pollack I, *et al.* Relapse from safer sex: the next challenge for AIDS prevention efforts. *Journal of Acquirred Immune Deficiency Syndromes* 1990; 3:1181–1187.
40. Dobs AS, Dempsey MA, Ladenson PW, Polk BF. Endocrine disorders in men infected with human immunodeficiency virus. *American Journal of Medicine* 1993; 84:611–615.
41. Tindall B, Forde S, Goldstein B, Ross MW. Sexual dysfunction in advanced HIV disease. *AIDS Care* 1994; 6:1:105–107.
42. Meyer-Bahlburg H, Exner TM, Lorenz G, *et al.* Sexual risk behavior, sexual functioning, and HIV-disease progression in gay men. *Journal of Sex Research* 1991; 28:3–27.
43. Bell A, Weinberg M. *Homosexualities—A Study of Diversity Among Men and Women*. New York: Simon and Schuster, 1978.
44. Rolland J. In sickness and in health; the impact of illness on couples' relationships. *Journal of Marital and Family Therapy* 1994; 20:327–347.
45. Doll LS, Byers RH, Bolan G, *et al.* Gay men who engage in high-risk sexual behavior. A multi-center comparison. *Sexually Transmitted Diseases* 1991; 18(3):170–175.
46. Powell-Cope GM. The experiences of gay couples affected by HIV infection. *Qualitative Health Research* 1995; 5:36–62.
47. Wardlaw LA. Sustaining informal caregivers for person with AIDS. Families in Society. *Journal of Contemporary Human Services* 1994; 75:373–384.
48. Folkman S, Chesney M, Christopher-Richards A. Stress and coping in caregiving partners of men with AIDS. *Psychiatric Clinics of North America* 1994; 1:35–53.
49. Mattison AM, McWhirter DP. Serodiscordant male couples. *Journal of Gay and Lesbian Social Services* 1994; 83–98.
50. Remien RH. Couples of serodisconcordant HIV status: Challenges and strategies for intervention with couples. In: Wicks, LA, ed. *Psychotherapy and AIDS: The Human Dimension*. Washington D.C.: Taylor & Francis; 1997; 167–179.
51. Berger RM. Men together: Understanding the gay couple. *Journal of Homosexuality* 1990; 19(3): 31–49.
52. Bosga MB, de Wit JBF, de Vroome EMM, *et al.* Differences in perception of risk for HIV infection with steady and non-steady partners among gay men. *AIDS Education and Prevention* 1995; 7(2): 103–115.
53. Henriksson B. Risk factor love. Homosexuality, sexual interaction and HIV prevention. Doctorial dissertation, University of Gothenburg, Sweden; 1995.
54. McLean J, Boulton M, Brookes D, *et al.* Regular partners and risky behavior: Why do gay men have unprotected intercourse? *AIDS Care* 1994; 6(3):331–341.
55. Becker S, Clement U. HIV infektion und AIDS. In: Im Uexkul, ed. *Psychosomatische Medizin*. 4 Auflage. München: Urben und Schwarzenberg 1990; 889–902.
56. Remien RH, Carballo-Dieguez A, Wagner G. Intimacy and sexual risk behavior in serodiscordant male couples. *AIDS Care* 1995; 7:429–438.
57. Odet W. *In the Shadow of the Epidemic. Being HIV-Negative in the Age of AIDS*. Durham, N.C.: Duke University Press; 1995.
58. Shelby RD. *People with HIV and Those Who Help Them. Challenges, Integration, Intervention*. New York: Harrington Park Press; 1995.

5

The Insidious Persecutory Drama of HIV

In this chapter, we will adopt a more finely grained look at the HIV scenario and those psychological issues that are evoked by the various HIV-related threats. The point of departure is the qualitative analysis of Dr. Schönnesson's psychotherapeutic notes of the 38 gay men with HIV. The most salient HIV-related psychological issues are portrayed in the light of the constructs of persecution, death anxiety, existential death anxiety and awareness, loss and mourning, control, despair versus hope, and psychological defenses. Table 2 illustrates that different psychological issues and the defenses occur with different intensity over the four disease phases (asymptomatic, mild symptomatic, severe symptomatic, and terminal).

PSYCHOLOGICAL ISSUES

Persecution

As described in Chapter 4, people with HIV live more or less constantly under threats toward their physical, sexual, and social existences. These in turn evoke a variety of emotions, cause worries, and may also induce emotional stress. Another way to view HIV-related threats and their concomitant emotions and worries is in terms of the concepts of external and internal persecutors. The latter will be highlighted in Chapter 9, as the internal persecutors intrude into the individual's self and integrity.

The individual with HIV has been and still is "attacked" by an external, alien, bad object—the virus. It persecutes and threatens an individual physically with death and annihilation. Medication and other medical treatments are also potentially perceived as persecutors, as they have an aggressive, intrusive character. Leo phrased it in the following way: "All these pills are poisoned and sooner or later they will kill me." But there are also "secondary" persecutors in terms of potential psychological, sexual, and social limitations. HIV-preventive campaigns that put all the responsibility on the person with HIV and the potential stigmatizing environment may be perceived as external "secondary" persecutors.

Table 2. HIV-Related Psychological Issues and Defenses over the Four HIV Disease Phases

	The asymptomatic phase	The mild symptomatic phase	The severe symptomatic phase	The terminal phase
Persecution	**Latent in terms of threat and worries**	**Manifest**	**Manifest; Non-escapable**	**Latent in terms of worries and fear**
Death	**Death anxiety, death wishes; Existential death awareness in terms of restriction of sex, life, and time**	**Death and existential death anxiety; Existential death awareness in terms of restriction of sex, intimacy, life, and time**	**Death anxiety; Manifest existential death awareness; Existential death awareness in terms of restriction of intimacy, life and time; Existential death anxiety; Death symbols**	**Death anxiety; Manifest existential death awareness; Existential death anxiety; Death symbols; Ambivalence; Resignation**
Loss, grief, mourning	Sexuality; Friends	**Sexuality; The body; Friends; Life; Fatherhood**	**Sexuality; The body; Friends; Life; Identity**	**Sexuality; The body; Life; Identity**
Loss of control	**Uncertainty**	**Uncertainty; Out of control**	**Uncertainty; Out of control**	**Uncertainty; Out of control**
Despair versus hope	Helplessness; Hopelessness; Despair	Vulnerability; Helplessness; Hopelessness; Despair; Hope	**Vulnerability; Helplessness; Hopelessness; Despair; Hope**	**Vulnerability; Helplessness; Hopelessness; Despair; Hope**
Defense strategies	Denial; Avoidance; Magical thinking	Denial; Avoidance; Magical thinking; Projection	Avoidance; Magical thinking; Projection	Avoidance; Magical thinking; Projection

Note: The bolded words indicate that the issues are particularly salient in that disease phase.

The qualitative analysis revealed that the persecutory theme unfolded over the four disease phases but was experienced differently depending upon the phase. In the asymptomatic phase the persecutor theme was expressed latently in terms of a sense of being threatened by and worried about HIV. Some of the men stated that their "life is threatened," whereas others felt threatened in their physical and sexual existences. Others expressed their worries "of becoming sick" or that they were "worried about the disease." One's own HIV-related worries and concerns can also be projected onto one's partner (or friends), for example, the statement "I'm so worried about my partner's health status" (projection does not exclude a genuine concern about one's partner's health status). Taken together, the persecutory theme was experienced in an insidious mode in the asymptomatic phase.

In the mild symptomatic phase, the physical threats changed into manifest experiences of being persecuted by HIV: "I'm persecuted by HIV"; "HIV has started to move around in my body." Some of those men who were engaged within the HIV movement talked about a general, almost overwhelming sense of persecution in that they were "surrounded by disease and death and there is no escape." As the infection starts to become real, concrete, and visible in the mild symptomatic phase, it is not surprising that the manifest persecutor scenario enters this disease phase. Gerald states: "HIV has caught up with me."

The experience of being exposed to the HIV persecutor, together with a feeling of not being able to escape from it, was salient in the severe symptomatic phase. Medication, and if there was an implanted port-a-cath, contributed to these feelings. Some men expressed very strong emotions like "scared to death" and "I dread the horror." In this disease phase some of the men talked about their "fear of reality." The fear and the persecutor scenario have indeed a realistic tone as the individual's health seriously started to deteriorate.

In the terminal phase the manifest sense of persecution subsides and is replaced with feelings of worries and fear. Common remarks are: "It is just going downhill"; "I'm so scared of becoming even sicker"; "What will happen to me?" Here, like in the previous disease phase, these statements are indeed realistic. HIV has succeeded in its persecution. Again, the individual is confronted with worries and uncertainty, but this time the worries are related to when the ultimate consequence—death—will enter his life.

Death Anxiety

According to Langs[1] there are two basic forms of death awareness; death as a physical or a psychological danger to life (predatory threats) and death as an existential fact. Both forms evoke death anxiety. The predatory threats evoke predatory death anxiety and the existential form arouses existential death anxiety. The latter refers to "the recognition of the inevitability of death for oneself and other humans and living creatures"[1] (p. 12) and fear of annihilation.

Death anxiety is not only aroused by death of loved ones or one's own impending death. It is also evoked by manifest death-related physical predatory events such as disease and injury (that bring up the possibility of death). Loss, separation, and emotional abandonment consciously or unconsciously arouse psychological death anxiety. Within the clinical setting we have to be alert to direct and indirect signs of activated physical or psychological death anxiety. Direct signs include direct allusions to death and its related themes and usually the manifest expression about death concerns and death anxiety, But death anxiety can also be expressed indirectly. The individual's emphasis on boundaries and finitude is an example of a subtle, indirect expression of death-related concerns and anxiety.

The qualitative analysis revealed that physical, psychological, and existential death-related themes and issues were of vital concern to the men during the whole course of the disease process. They approached the themes and issues in both a direct and an indirect way as described below.

Physical Death Anxiety

In all four disease phases the men expressed their physical death anxiety. Quite common direct statements are: "I'm afraid to die"; "I'm afraid of death"; "I'm afraid to slowly languish"; "I dread death." Others relate death anxiety to waiting: "It is an eternal awaiting of death"; or "HIV is like being killed gradually." Still other men addressed their death anxiety indirectly in terms of being afraid of the AIDS diagnosis, their friends' death, or their psychological pain in saying good-bye. Thoughts about funeral, cremation, or the will also evoked death anxiety among some of the men. Another manifestation of death anxiety was the experience that it is "impossible to give in." It was not uncommon to hear exclamations of not wanting to die or that the individual is "not allowed" to die because of their partner or parents or hospital staff. In the severe symptomatic and terminal phases, death and death anxiety were also expressed symbolically as sharks, boats, and long tunnels.

The other side of the coin, longing for death and longing to die in peace, was brought up mainly in the asymptomatic and the severe symptomatic disease phases. In the asymptomatic phase the individual is very much confronted with uncertainty of the disease, and the wish for dying could be a "solution" to shortcut the disease process. In the severe symptomatic phase, when HIV-related symptoms are reality, the longing for death could be understood as an "enough is enough" attitude; the end to physical and psychological suffering is long overdue.

The dying process. Death encompasses two meanings: dying—the process leading up to death—and death in the sense of not existing.[2] Death is an unknown state as no one has returned from death and been able to tell us about it. Dying, on the contrary, is a process and is related to past and future time. Usually we think of dying as a period when the person has a particular disease or is in a particular phase of a disease that usually leads to death. In the case of HIV the dying period is sometimes difficult to assess. Some of the men Dr. Schönnesson has met have been diagnosed as "dying" but in some miraculous way returned to life. Afterward they have expressed feelings of being cheated. Jeffrey comments:

> I had prepared myself to die—and then I don't. I am furious. Now I have to go through the whole process again. And how can I be sure that I actually do die next time?

Dying is not merely a biological/medical process but also a psychological process.[2] Efforts have been made to systematize dying into stages. Kübler-Ross's five-stage process of dying[3]—denial, anger, bargaining, depression, and acceptance—is probably the most cited one. But her division into stages is nowadays questioned. First, not all people who are dying follow these stages in a sequence and second they are not typical of every dying person. Others'[4] experiences as well as Dr. Schönnesson's are that alternation and oscillation between different forms of emotions and reactions characterize dying. Among people who are dying we recognize ambivalence between clinging to life (the will to live) and yearning for peace and an end (the desire to die). We quite often observe that gay men who are terminally ill with HIV show this psychic splitting. In this splitting two opposite ideas are verbalized; one in which the close death is fully realized and one in which the idea is distinguished by the faith in surviving, often depicted in vivid fantasies about the future. William, for example, applied for admission to a university three weeks prior to his death. Peter bought a new puppy in the month before he died. The psychic splitting, which is also found in other terminal diseases, facilitates the man's acceptance of his impending death and helps him to withstand death fear. From a professional perspective this split communicates irrationality and goes against our understanding of reality. However, Dreifuss-Kattan[4] emphasizes that professionals have to accept this split otherwise they are of no use to the dying person. It is only when the professional can deal simultaneously with both parts that the dying person feels "contained as a whole person who can receive love for both his surviving and dying parts"[4] (p. 102). Within such an attitudinal framework, the dying person is regarded as a living person until he dies.

We can also see how dying people oscillate between acceptance and denial of death. According to Feigenberg, fluctuations in the balance between acceptance and denial are not only the effects of the individual's psychological makeup and the process of dying, but also "the person who happens to be communicating with him"[2] (p. 24). Family members, in particular, were perceived by some of the men as "obstacles" to keep them from dying. Arthur reflected: "Mom doesn't want me to die—although I'm ready to go. So I have to pretend to her that I won't die, but I know I'll very soon."

Another aspect of death anxiety is the fear of dying. It is a fear of being overtaken by HIV that is to persecute and ultimately consume the person. The terminal phase of the HIV disease is the peak of long-term uncertainties. It incorporates "the loss of everything that human life contains. The dying person must mourn everything he knows and loves, and he does not know what to expect in their place"[4] (p. 89). The person usually conveys an ambivalent attitude toward death and is fearful of abandonment and painful dying. A sense of being abandoned increases when family members are unwilling or unable to acknowledge the impending death of the person. He then has to deal with his death anxiety and other death-related issues on his own. On the other hand forcing the person to discuss his impending death may also cause emotional discomfort. At this stage, the person knows he is dying and he usually does not want to talk about dying and death as that brings him closer to death and the inevitable. In the later modes of dying most people withdraw into themselves and detach from life realities. They feel more and more lonely in their impending death as there is no stand-in for or companion in one's death. However, fantasies can be of some comfort. Kevin often shared with the therapist his fear of physical and psychological death and "the bridge to the other side" fantasy.

> You know that I am afraid of dying. But if you are there on the other side then I am not afraid any more. Please promise me that you won't abandon me.

The fantasy is also a reflection of how important it is as a therapist to strive for meeting the mirroring, twinship, and idealizing needs of the vulnerable dying person. As Kohut states:

> A human death can and, I will affirm, should be an experience that, however deeply melancholy, is comparable to a fulfilled parting—it should have no significant admixture of disintegration anxiety. It must be stressed, however, that in order to enable the dying person to retain a modicum of the cohesion, firmness, and harmony of the self, his surroundings must not withdraw their selfobject functions [mirroring, twinship, idealization] at the last moment of his conscious participation in the world.[5] (p. 18)

Toward the end of his life, Leonard often fell asleep for a longer or shorter period of time during the therapeutic sessions in his home. He said:

> it's great to wake up having you here at my bedside. It also feels good when you wake me up. In that way I can postpone the sleep and later on I can get a 100% out of it.

Indirectly his "naps" can be seen as "a rehearsal of dying." He needed to do so in order to lessen his death anxiety. But Leonard also wanted to make sure that the therapist's psychological support continued while he was asleep and that it was available after he woke up. This experience comforted him in his dying process and protected him from experiencing disintegration anxiety.

In the dying phase, the person knows he is dying and therefore there is no comfort for him in talking about it. Thus, silence becomes the language within the therapeutic context. It is more important being there and listening rather than talking. The experienced losses can also be compensated for by "experiencing together" with the therapist, such as listening to music or the therapist reading from a book. Dr. Schönnesson had worked with Steven for nearly six years and now she was accompanying him in his final stage of life. During the last five months he had been in and out of the hospital and his health dramatically deteriorated. Steven suffered from brain disease causing him difficulties in talking and he was partly immobilized. In their sessions the therapist often had to help him hold the glass of water or to feed him when he so wished. The twice or three times a week sessions followed the same procedure. Steven wanted the therapist to sit in the same chair at the same spot at his bedside and then they listened to a classical piece of music—usually a piano or a violin piece. One day he asked her to bring him books of which he would choose one for the therapist to read to him. "What kinds of books?" she asked him. Steven answered, "You know which books I like, and take them from your home." So the therapist brought along some books and Steven chose *Siddhartha* by Herman Hesse. They continued their routine of first listening to a piece of music and then she read from the book. Steven decided how much the therapist should read. He became more and more apprehensive about her leaving him. She had to "warn" him as time was drawing toward its end of the session. This very special session Steven asked the therapist to sit down on his bed. He sat up in the bed. At this stage he could hardly speak. She wore a long-sleeved blouse and he pulled up the sleeves to the elbows, took her arms and placed them around his knees and then putting his bare arms around hers. They were both silent looking into each other's eyes. After a while Steven lay down, closed his eyes, and said "Music and read." And so the therapist did. She read the last chapter in *Siddhartha*. Then he asked her to write down in his calendar their next meeting. He got angry with the therapist for not writing it down in hers, so she took up the calendar and made a note. She showed it to him and he said "Good." Two days later Steven died.

In this last session, both knew that Steven was close to death. Just like Leonard, Steven tried to anticipate his death through a kind of rehearsal. In his fantasy, Steven merged with the therapist by means of the body contact in an illusion that he would not have to be alone in death. Steven's wish to listen to music while the therapist read from the book is another merger fantasy. But this union scenario also communicated a strong desire that she hold him close and protectively. At the same time, Steven protected himself—and probably even the therapist—from a complete fusion by not having her hold him in her arms. In this way, Steven showed autonomy.

Dreifuss-Kattan[4] notes that a growing weakness because of the disease may facilitate the person's adaptation to impending death. "A dying man needs to die, as a sleepy man needs to sleep, and there comes a time when it is wrong, as well as useless, to resist"[6] (p. 91).

Psychological Death Anxiety

There seems to be some similarities between Langs' psychological death anxiety and Kohut's disintegration anxiety.[5] Disintegration anxiety refers to fear of loss of humanness, that is, a fear of psychological death. Kohut emphasizes that it is not fear of loss of love that is at stake here but the individual fears loosing the mirroring, twinship, and idealized functions of people in his environment. Without this "psychological oxygen" the self cannot psychologically survive and ultimately ceases to be a human self.

The qualitative data showed that fear of psychological death was of concern to the men, in particular during the mild symptomatic phase. The fear was related to becoming dependent, nonhuman, or invisible, to being abandoned, rejected, forgotten, or disclosed. When the individual enters this disease phase, HIV becomes real and he becomes aware of the potential social and psychological consequences of the infection. The fear of psychological death is shared with people who have been diagnosed with cancer, but there is the difference of stigmatization between the two diseases. Among people with HIV, the stigmatized status of HIV/AIDS reinforces the psychological death anxiety. Some of the men who were in their terminal phase of the HIV disease experienced psychological death in that friends or family rejected them or they felt forgotten by their friends. Others expressed a sense of being "a living dead person" because of brain lesions. Common remarks were: "I don't recognize myself any longer"; "I just exist but I don't live"; "I'm no one."

Existential Death Awareness and Existential Death Anxiety

Existential death awareness came to the forefront in all disease phases and existential death anxiety in all but the first one. The latter, the fear of annihilation, was phrased as "I'm scared to languish," "everything is darkness and chaos," "the thought of cremation scares me to death," "HIV suffocates me," "life is flowing out of me." Some men also conveyed their sense of psychological annihilation, which was manifested in their experience of being sexually and intimately obliterated.

Existential death awareness of the inevitable death was approached in terms of "I'm mortal" and "I'm going to die." In the terminal phase of life there appeared to be an oscillation between the realization of being mortal and the sense of being immortal. Some of the men also showed an ambivalent attitude toward death in this disease phase; on the one hand there was a longing for death "to get peace" and on the other hand a longing for life. Another characteristic of the terminal phase was a sense of resignation. To some men it was reflected in words like "it's soon over" and "I'm ready to die soon." Others "want to give in," whereas others meant "there is nothing left to live for." "It's time to give in now" and "it's over now" are other examples of resignation.

A common theme among the men was their experiences of restrictions and boundaries. From an existential perspective we would argue that the theme is an indirect (and probably unconscious) manifestation of existential death awareness in that boundaries are equivalent to finitude or death. The men talked about sexual, time, and life ("life is tightened") restrictions in the asymptomatic phase. They in turn fostered a sense of being encapsulated and in despair, "everything is too late now."

The mild symptomatic phase was characterized by a sense of boundaries related to time, life, sexuality, and intimacy. Some of the men also experienced and expressed their "lost fatherhood." Many of them conveyed their sense of being imprisoned and in despair and pain in acknowledging the restrictions of life and time, as exemplified by the following quotes: "I simply can't deny HIV any longer and that hurts"; "I can't run away any longer but I have to face reality"; "It is terrible to know that there isn't enough time."

Medical treatments and HIV-related symptoms in the severe symptomatic phase were experienced by the men as restricting time, life, and intimacy. "HIV restricts my possibilities of finding a partner"; "My time has its ending"; "Time is short"; "The boundaries of my life are obvious." These restrictions in turn fostered a sense of being confined and imprisoned as well as being violated.

In the terminal phase, the men expressed a realization of the finitude of their lives as in the words of Tom and David:

> There isn't much time left now.
>
> There is no turning back.

Summary

In the asymptomatic disease phase death concerns were related to death anxiety and longing for death. Indirectly, the men talked about death in terms of sexual, time, and life restrictions, which fostered a sense of being encapsulated and in despair.

Death and existential death anxieties, senses of time, life, sexual and intimacy boundaries characterized the mild symptomatic phase. Some of the men also experienced and expressed their "lost fatherhood." Many of them conveyed their sense of being imprisoned, in despair and pain in acknowledging the restrictions of life and time.

In the severe symptomatic and terminal phases death issues were reflected in death anxiety, existential death awareness and death anxiety, as well as death symbols. In the severe symptomatic phase the men experienced being restricted in time, life, and intimacy, and these restrictions furthered a sense of being confined and imprisoned as well as being insulted. Men in the terminal phase tended to bring up issues related to ambivalence and resignation as well as avoidance of death thoughts. They also expressed a realization of the finitude of their lives.

Loss, Grief, and Mourning

In the course of the HIV disease the person will be faced with multiple losses, which cause psychological pain manifested in grief and mourning. Mourning in turn produces feelings of pain, loss of interest in an outside world perceived as miserable and empty, and loss of capacity to reach out for others. The latter is a paradox as reconnection with one's social network is important to mourning. Grief can be seen as a state of tension between presence and absence, that is, living with a present absence.[7] It is often regarded as something taxing with negative connotation, whereas its healing dimensions are often forgotten or overlooked. Grief can lead to change through the mourning process. It faces four challenges in a circular course: acknowledgment of losses, release of emotions related to grief, acquiring new skills to regain trust in life, and reinvestment of energy from the past to the present.[8] In addition, the mourning process is a reflection of both the kind of loss the individual has experienced and the internal meaning of the loss to the bereaved. Sometimes grief can be of such a magnitude and the individual has such minimal access to his psychological and social resources that he ends up in a "frozen" state of grief. It can for example be reflected in the individual's reluctance to engage, or difficulties in engaging, in new relationships. There is a fear of being abandoned again or that the individual himself may cause his partner grief through his own death. Under more favorable conditions, grief can be an essential part of personal development and maturity.[7]

Persons with HIV experience multiple HIV-related losses and consequently many mourning processes as well. The losses are not only related to their own person but also to losses of loved ones and acquaintances, that is, a massive bereavement.[9] The interpersonal losses are to some of the men a salient theme during the disease process, except in the terminal phase. They grieve for their dying or dead friends and some of them also express survival guilt: "He had been sick for a much shorter time than I so why he and not me?"

The qualitative analysis of the psychotherapeutic notes revealed, however, that most experienced losses were related to the person himself. The loss of one's sexuality was a reoccurring theme regardless of disease phase, "Sex isn't there any more for me." Such a statement and similar ones were also an expression of losing one's gay lifestyle (and its associated social support and subcultural identification) that many men grew up taking for granted. This includes homosexual courtship, mating, and lovemaking rituals.[10] O'Leary[10] points out that those gay men with an HIV-negative status experience a loss of status from a marginally accepted group to an even lower one within society. The same holds true for gay men with HIV, but they also perceive a similar drop in status within the gay subcultures. Another aspect of sexuality is the theme of lost fatherhood, in particular in the mild symptomatic phase. Robert says: "Now being HIV positive all my chances to become a father are gone. Earlier—before I got HIV—I still had the possibility if I had wanted."

Gay men with HIV, just the same as people with cancer,[4] mourn the losses of the illusionary timelessness, body parts and functions, identity, and life itself. These losses found their voice directly and indirectly. Examples of direct expressions are statements like: "It is damn hard not to be able to live like before"; "I'm deteriorating"; "I'm loosing my human dignity"; "I am loosing myself"; "I have lost my life"; "I'm loosing everything." Indirectly the perceived time and life boundaries, as discussed earlier, are also manifestations of losses that have to be mourned.

Closely linked to loss is the concept of separation. To lose someone or something always includes separation, to say good-bye and to mourn, which is usually psychologically painful. In the phase of dying, ties to significant others have to be broken, fostering grief, despair, anxiety, and guilt. Norman states: "It is so terribly painful to say good-bye to my partner and family. But I have to express the words 'good-bye' to die in peace." Tom on the other hand said his good-byes internally and concluded, "Now I can die in peace and harmony."

Control

The individual's struggle over control (or power) issues becomes more pronounced along the disease progression, as he faces more and more physical loss of control. It can easily carry over into anxiety over potential loss of control of the self, as HIV (like cancer) is often experienced as a threat to one's self or identity.[11] These aspects of control were prominent themes over the HIV disease process and in particular in the severe symptomatic phase. The qualitative analysis indicated that the sense of loss of control was in particular related to a loss of control of the self as reflected in quotes like, "I have no control whatsoever"; "There is nothing I can do." But it also happened that the physical loss of control came to the surface: "I'm in the claws of HIV"; "I have lost control of HIV and time and that's scary." Most of the men talked about the aspect of uncertainty, a paraphrase of loss of control. Its consuming feeling is exemplified in the statement: "I'm eaten up by uncertainty."

Persons who experience loss of control try in various ways to regain their control. Empirical data show, for example, that active involvement in one's health and self-efficacy increases one's sense of being in control and the degree of one's resilience.[12,13] The qualitative analysis of the psychotherapeutic notes clearly brought out that the gay men needed to be in control of HIV. On one level they do know that there is no way to master the virus, but by means of defense strategies the individual may perceive an illusionary control. At the same time it is psychologically life sustaining to identify (in this case) HIV-related domains over which there is a realistic chance to practice control and in that way to reduce the risk of feeling powerlessness and helplessness.

In their endeavor for control, the gay men employed various strategies, such as cognitive-physical, existential, and defense strategies. These strategies are in general in the service of adaptation and an attempt to organize and control the experience. Whereas the existential and the defense strategies were present in all disease phases, cognitive-physical strategies were employed in all phases except the asymptomatic one. The cognitive dimension of the latter strategies was manifested in the efforts to keep up with the latest news about HIV and medication and to take an active part in decisions regarding one's medication and other medical treatments. An example of the physical dimension of the cognitive-physical strategy was to be alert to physical changes—even minor ones—and discuss them with the physician. Roger states. "I want to be in 100% control of my body."

Existential strategies were reflected in the individual's need to be in control of his funeral by preparing it. Hubert is a spokesman of the gay men in saying: "I want to be in charge here, so I know that it really goes the way I want it." It was also important to many of the men to write their will. Thoughts about suicide and a sense of having the freedom to choose suicide "if worst comes to worst" provided them with control as expressed by Simon and Adam:

> "I have the right to decide when to give in."
>
> "I want to control death."

The illusionary control, regardless of disease phase, is manifested in the defense strategy of magical thinking. Some men argued that if they "behave well" or "take really good care of myself" or if "I move to this city" would protect them from HIV. Others felt that as long as they were in psychotherapy or engaged in the HIV movement that HIV would not attack them. William states his magical thinking in the following way: "I've made a pact with HIV."

Despair versus Hope

When a person's very being is threatened by death and his control of what is happening to him gradually decreases, he may employ a spectrum of reactions including vulnerability, helplessness, and hopelessness turning into despair. According to the *American College Dictionary*, despair refers to "the loss of hope in regard to a particular situation." The qualitative analysis implied that regardless of disease phase, there was an undercurrent sense of despair. Although the gay men along the whole disease process expressed these reactions, they were more salient in the severe symptomatic and terminal phases of the HIV disease. In the asymptomatic phase, the men expressed more of a general sense of despair. Sometimes it was voiced in terms of despair over friends dying, which also could be interpreted as a projection of despair over oneself into others.

Feelings of vulnerability, hopelessness, and helplessness were reflected in the mild and severe symptomatic phases. Vulnerability was expressed in words as: "I'm so vulnerable and defenseless," and hopelessness as: "I'm a hopeless case"; "There is no hope for me." The sense of helplessness was manifested in quotes like: "No one can protect me from HIV"; "The health care system can't help me"; "Nothing can save me." In the terminal phase, the sense of hopelessness, helplessness, and despair was more often talked about in direct association to the disease:

"It is horrible to realize how very sick and helpless I am"; "There is so much despair in me because I have lost so much."

Feelings of loss of control, hopelessness, helplessness, and despair are concomitant with depression and are supposed to be a necessary phase of the working-through process.[4] The concept of depression is often loosely used and has both a popular and a psychiatric meaning. Judd notes: "The popular use describes a frequent occurrence, is a part of normal existence, and is not an illness. The psychiatric term may have features of an illness, depending on its severity"[14] (p. 69). Winnicott summarizes the phenomenon (cited in Judd):

> Depression belongs to psychopathology. It can be severe and crippling and may last a lifetime, and it is commonly a passing mood in relatively healthy individuals. At the normal end, depression, which is a common, almost universal, phenomenon, related to mourning, to the capacity to feel guilt, and to the maturational process.[14] (p. 69)

Winnicott's description of depression as relating to mourning implies that it is a "normal" response to the abnormal situation of being confronted by a life-threatening illness. Although we agree with Winnicott's perspective we would recommend making use of the concept of depressive mood in order to keep the necessary and important distinction from clinical depression.

The psychotherapeutic notes of the gay men clearly portrayed that whereas clinical depression was rare, depressive mood was common, albeit intermittently, in particular in the severe symptomatic and terminal phases. The depressive mood usually was manifested in a sense of hopelessness, helplessness, and despair. When depressive mood appears within the HIV disease scenario, it signals that it is no longer possible to escape the perceived HIV persecutor but the individual has to admit, "I am suffering from HIV." In other words, the defense of denial can no longer protect the individual from the HIV reality.

The sense of helplessness, which results in hopelessness, describes an absence of hope. The *American College Dictionary* defines hopelessness as "a feeling of futility and passive abandonment of oneself to fate." Judd[14] emphasizes that hope and despair cannot be felt simultaneously, but there has to be an oscillation between the two. Hope, which is an abstract term, is future-oriented and related to achieve something better. Hope, according to Erikson, is one of the vital values of life: "Hope is the enduring belief in the attainability of fervent wishes"[15] (p. 256). Further, he argues that hope is a reflection of basic trust; those who have basic trust also have hope. A similar approach is suggested by Feigenberg,[2] in which hope is assumed to rest on a sense of and a confidence in being welcome and wanted. Labonté[16] argues that the sense of hope presumably derives from a sense of being in control. However, meaning of hope differs between individuals and may vary during different times and circumstances of our lives.[17]

Within any disease scenario, there is a need to keep in touch with hope and hopefulness. Too often though, hope refers solely to the cure of the disease or longevity. Within the HIV realm the cure perspective is—for the present at least—

unlikely, although one significant subset of hope is the hope for a medical breakthrough. On the other hand, people who are symptomatic may experience hopefulness in terms of having certain HIV-related symptoms cured. Those who are on combination treatment may face the possibility of having HIV-related symptoms postponed and thus to live longer without symptoms.

However, Nuland points out that within a severe disease scenario, hope could be redefined:

> There are those who will find hope in faith and their belief in an afterlife; some will look forward to the moment a milestone is reached or a deed is accomplished; there are even some whose hope is centered on maintaining the kind of control that will permit them the means to decide the moment of their death; ... Whatever form it may take, each of us find hope in his or her own way.[17] (p. 257)

Over one-half of the men in the course of their psychotherapy mentioned a sense of hopefulness. To some men hope was about the wish to be remembered after their death; to others hope referred to medical treatment. However, mostly the men talked about hope in an unspecified manner like, "There is still hope for me" or "I feel hopeful." Although it was infrequently brought up, hope was most salient in the severe symptomatic and the terminal phase. Data also showed that the men were more inclined to talk about hope at the end of the psychotherapeutic work—either self-terminated or by death—in comparison to the beginning of the psychotherapeutic contact. This change could be a reflection of the men's sense that their initial subjective helplessness was or is on its way to be undercut in favor of their abilities to be self-assertive and to take actions for themselves and about themselves.[11] Another interpretation—of an existential character—is that the person realizes that he has the possibility to make his choices in life. He does not have to live in symbiosis with HIV. For example, one man concluded that he did not have to restrict his life to the triangle of the hospital, our center, and the body positive group, but that he was free to expand his life space. That insight infused him with hope.

As clinicians, we face the paradox of empathy and hopelessness. We are expected to be empathic toward, supportive of, and hope providers for the person with HIV. On the other hand we are aware of the significance of hopelessness, when it comes to the HIV-infection itself, as we cannot cure it. However, we can offer the person the hope that we are there to share, contain and hold his loss and grief, suffering, pain, hopelessness, and despair; but also joy and happiness; in other words the hope to be acknowledged, seen, and respected as a whole human being.

Psychological Defenses

People living with HIV, like people diagnosed with cancer, are confronted with a mixture of fears that derive from various sources such as reality-based fears, fantasy-based fears, and death anxiety. In their strivings for not being overwhelmed by fears and other emotions, people protect themselves by means of psychological defenses. Among the gay men, denial and projection were common employed defenses across the disease process.

Denial

Denial is an effort to cope with anxiety associated with the threat to life and it mutes distress, at least temporarily.[4] Adaptive denial does not mean that the individual does not recognize that he is sick but rather adopts a positive attitude toward the outcome of the infection. Jeffrey was assertive in his conviction that: "I'll be the first person to combat HIV." Denial is also a function of a deep belief in one's inviolability.[18] Once the defense of denial is undermined and the individual really grasps that he is going to die "like all the others," he feels lost and "betrayed."

Denial can take the form of a conscious attempt to forget, deny, and avoid thinking of HIV. Another form is repression, which is an unconscious process in which painful or unaccepted HIV-related thoughts or feelings are prevented from coming to consciousness. To some this defense is necessary in order to go on living and to cope with new life conditions. Clinical experiences in general show that when denial persists or increases during the disease process, the individual splits off all feelings linked to suffering and pain. "This denial requires psychological help and should not be supported by the doctor or treatment team as it often is"[4] (p. 64). The most common pattern is for the individual to develop gradually a more selective denial directed to particular aspects of the disease.

People who deny their HIV infection do so not only to protect themselves from painful emotions and thoughts, but denial also has a social function, in that it is meant to keep significant others in good spirits and thus prevent their withdrawal. It is plausible that denial is employed to a higher degree by gay men diagnosed with HIV than with other diseases or nongay people with HIV, since they are doubly stigmatized (gayness and HIV) and thus constantly under the threat of being shunned by others.

Projection

Projection refers to a defense strategy in which the individual puts unbearable painful or offensive emotions or thoughts onto another person. In that way the painful emotions are perceived in another person instead of within oneself. However, when the individual projects his negative feelings he runs the risk of perceiving his environment as hostile and bad, and he may feel attacked and devalued. For example, some gay men in Dr. Schönnesson's case load projected their feelings of hopelessness onto health staff, who were then perceived as not doing their best and not being there for the person. This in turn reinforced the sense of helplessness and hopelessness that may be projected onto others, and a vicious circle is at hand. Another example is when the person projects his death anxiety onto others, who then are perceived as "bad" in that "they do not allow me to die." On the other hand this can indeed be a realistic perception of significant others who have great difficulties in themselves to accept death.

Almost any aspect of HIV can evoke aggression that is a disguised manifestation of feelings of helplessness and hopelessness in the face of HIV. Other examples than those mentioned above that the gay men brought up were the sense of being controlled by HIV, medication, hospital staff, significant others, all which evoked aggression or rage. Aggression can also be a manifestation of envy. People with HIV, like people with cancer, may experience envy toward healthy people who are free to come and go and behave as they want. However, aggression is another perceived "negative" emotion that often engenders projection. The target of aggressive outbursts is often hospital staff or significant others who do not respond to the person's needs for empathy and sensitivity.

> The patient's expectations are thus disappointed, and his fragile sense of self-worth is again badly injured; the ensuing outbursts is an expression of pent-up narcissistic rage.[4] (p. 71)

REFERENCES

1. Langs R. *Death Anxiety and Clinical Practice.* London: Karnac Books; 1997.
2. Feigenberg L. *Terminal Care: Friendship Contracts with Dying Cancer Patients.* New York: Brunner & Mazel; 1980.
3. Kübler-Ross E. *On Death and Dying.* London: Tavistock; 1970.
4. Dreifuss-Kattan E. *Cancer Stories. Creativity and Self-Repair.* Hillsdale, N.J.: Analytic Press; 1990.
5. Kohut H. *How Does Psychoanalysis Cure?* Chicago: University of Chicago Press; 1984.
6. Alsop S as cited in Dreifuss-Kattan E. *Cancer Stories. Creativity and Self-Repair.* Hillsdale, N.J.: Analytic Press; 1990.
7. Kallenberg K, Bråkenhielm CR. Pain and suffering as existential questions in palliative care. *European Journal of Palliative Care* 1994; 1(1):54–56.
8. Davidsen-Nielsen M. *Bland lejon. Att leva med livshotande sjukdom.* Stockholm: Norstedts förlag; 1995.
9. Blechner MJ. Psychodynamic approaches to AIDS and HIV. In: Blechner MJ, ed. *Hope and Mortality. Psychodynamic Approaches to AIDS and HIV.* Hillsdale, N.J.: Analytic Press; 1997; 3–62.
10. O'Leary JV. A heterosexual male therapist's journey of self-discovery: Wearing a "straight" jacket in a gay men's bereavement group. In: Blechner MJ, ed. *Hope and Mortality. Psychodynamic Approaches to AIDS and HIV.* Hillsdale, N.J.: Analytic Press; 1997; 209–220.
11. Rennecker RE. Cancer and psychotherapy. In: Goldberg JG, ed. *Psychotherapeutic Treatment of Cancer Patients.* London: Transaction Publishers; 1990; 131–166.
12. Moulton JM, Sweet DM, Temoshok L. Understanding attributions and health behavior changes in AIDS and ARC. Implications for intervention. In Temoshok L, Baum A, eds. *Psychosocial*

Perspectives on AIDS Ethiology, Prevention, and Treatment. Hillsdale, N.J.: Lawrence Erlbaum; 1990; 191–200.
13. Rabkin J, Williams JBW, Neugebauer R, *et al.* Maintenance of hope in HIV-spectrum homosexual men. *American Journal of Psychiatry* 1990; 147(10):1322–1326.
14. Judd D. *Give Sorrow Words. Working with a Dying Child.* London: Whurt Publishers; 1996.
15. Erikson EH. *Insight and Responsibility*. New York: Norton; 1964.
16. Labonté R. Measurement and practice. Power issues in quality of life, health promotion, and empowerment. In: Remwick R, Brown I, Nagler M, eds. *Quality of Life in Health Promotion and Rehabilitation. Conceptual Approaches, Issues, and Applications*. London: Sage Publications; 1996; 132–145.
17. Nuland SB. *How We Die. Reflections on Life's Final Chapter*. New York: Vintage Books; 1993.
18. Yalom I. *Existential Psychotherapy*. New York: Basic Books; 1980.

6

The Impact of HIV Infection on Psychological Functioning and Quality of Life

The HIV-related physical, social, and sexual threats, as well as psychological issues discussed in previous chapters, represent profound threats to the individual's psychological well-being and quality of life. The threats and issues are stressful in that they are undesirable and involve psychological change, "for good or ill, or by return to the psychological status quo ante"[1] (p. 3). It should be remembered though that stress vulnerability might oscillate over time but also be selective; for example, an individual may be affected by sexual threats but less so by social threats.

In the first section of this chapter we focus on the impact of HIV-related threats on psychological functioning in terms of depression, suicide, mood distress, and grief from an individual as well as couple perspective. The influence of psychological and social mediators on psychological functioning is discussed in the second section, followed by a discussion of the quality of life issue. As in the previous chapters, clinical data here refer to Dr. Schönnesson's quantitative and qualitative analysis of her psychotherapeutic notes of gay men with HIV.

THE IMPACT OF HIV INFECTION ON PSYCHOLOGICAL FUNCTIONING

Some people appear to be minimally psychologically affected by their disease. Rabkin et al.[2] found in their study among long-term AIDS survivors that depression, anxiety, and hostility were mild and unrelated to physical impairment. However, a sense of hopelessness was related to the degree of physical impairment, although degree of hopelessness was mild too. Overall the emergent theme was that of psychological resilience and positive survival. Similar results were found in Rabkin et al.'s subsequent study[3] in that both gay men with HIV and uninfected men displayed high levels of hope and low levels of current depressive symptoms. The quantitative analysis of the psychotherapeutic notes also showed (as stated in Chapter 5) that hope was experienced by over one-half of the men.

Despite severe symptoms (phase 3), they expressed a resilient attitude. Neither anxiety, powerlessness, nor despair or hopelessness correlated with symptoms.

As will be illustrated in what follows, empirical and clinical data show that others may experience more or less intense psychological distress in the course of the disease. It is reflected on a spectrum from psychiatric disorders to transient mood symptoms. Whereas the vast majority of empirical research has focused on the impact of HIV disease as such, minimal research has specifically investigated the impact of physical, social, or sexual HIV-related stressors on psychological well-being and even less so on quality of life among gay men living with HIV. One exception is Thompson et al.'s study,[4] in which the participants identified stressors in the areas of relationships, finances, and the illness of others. In turn, these stressors were associated with more depression. Further, Thompson et al. found that the number of stressors was linked with more alcohol consumption and perceived stress (i.e., the emotional response to the stressor) was positively associated with more tobacco use and unprotected sexual behaviors. For the vast majority of the participants, the predominant unprotected sexual practice was oral sex without a condom. The researchers emphasize that whereas the men with HIV are potentially being exposed to sexually transmittable diseases by means of unprotected oral sex, "the vast majority of this group do not practice behaviors that are likely to put HIV-negative individuals at risk"[4] (p. 10).

Foci of research have to a large extent been on whether there are differences in distress between people with HIV and uninfected people or differences over disease phases. Depression in particular has received major attention.

Depression

Although clinical depression is the most common psychiatric diagnosis among gay men with HIV, it is urgent to emphasize that depression is not the norm. Several studies show elevated rates of lifetime depression, but the rates of current major depression are in the 5% to 9% range,[5–9] comparable to those presented by people with cancer.[10] There are indications that those who currently suffer from depression have had depressive episodes that antedate HIV infection.[11] If depression or other psychiatric symptoms occur in the later stages of the HIV disease in particular, it is important that the counselor/psychotherapist bears in mind that these symptoms can be a result of biological disease processes in the brain. On the other hand, it is not always easy to differentiate between psychological and biological causes, and there may also been an interaction between the two.

It is interesting to note in a historical perspective that in the very early days of the HIV epidemic, studies reported exceptionally high rates of clinical depression and anxiety among gay men with HIV.[12–14] Studies that are more recent, however, display another picture in that gay men with HIV and those who are noninfected are approximately equal in rates of depression and anxiety.[6,8,9,15,16] Clement et al.[17] demonstrate in their meta-analysis similar results.

The different findings between early and more recent studies may be explained in terms of methodological issues. In the early studies, data were based on self-report rating scales and the samples were recruited from medical settings. Later investigations rely more on community-based samples, and instruments that were used were symptom lists that were sometimes complemented with psychiatric diagnostic instruments. Yet one could also raise the question whether this change could also partly be a reflection of changes within the sociomedical context. The neglect, panic, despair, and "therapeutic impotence"[18] that very much characterized the first years of the HIV epidemic have changed into a more optimistic and less panic-stricken attitude. Today the sociomedical climate is characterized by a "perhaps premature therapeutic triumphalism."[18] These changes may be internalized on an individual level and fewer experience depression. Further, more is "known" about HIV and its process, and much of the original uncertainty has dissipated. A sense of greater control and knowledge may also decrease depression through the appearance of greater predictability.

There is a common belief that people with HIV must be depressed or at least develop a clinical depression when they approach death. Cross-sectional studies on gay men at different phases of the HIV infection yield inconsistent results on this matter. Some reports have found different rates of depression in samples at different stages of HIV illness,[19,20] whereas others have not.[2,7,9,15,21,22] However, Rabkin et al.[9] found an increase in chronic low-grade depression as HIV symptoms emerged and progressed. In another study, Rabkin et al. state that available evidence is inconclusive "about the prevalence of depression in the HIV illness and whether rates increase with progression"[23] (p. 232). In contrast, the meta-analytic study by Clement et al.[17] showed that depression increases as the disease progresses, perhaps as degrees of uncertainty decrease.

Our empirical knowledge is however sparse with respect to *longitudinal* changes in rates of depression. Existing follow-up data suggest that rates of depression do not increase over time despite HIV disease progression.[21,24,25] In Perry et al.'s[7] study there was a decline in depressive symptom severity over a one-year period. These studies did not demonstrate any depression rate differences between infected and uninfected gay men on any occasion. In contrast, Rabkin et al.[23] found that the gay men with HIV, compared with the HIV-negative men, tended to have higher rates of major depression, but the difference did not increase over time.

The quantitative analysis of the psychotherapeutic notes of the 38 gay men showed that eight (21%) of the men expressed depressive symptoms and therefore were referred to psychiatrists at the center. Two of these men were in the asymptomatic phase, four in the mild symptomatic phase, and one in the severe symptomatic and terminal disease phase respectively. Six of these men were diagnosed as clinically depressed, received anti-depressant medication, and recovered from the depression.

Interestingly enough, studies on depression do not provide any information regarding whether the participants have previously been or are currently in any kind of counseling or psychotherapy. This kind of information is important when it comes to interpretation of the data. It is plausible that a "resilient" attitude may be an artifact of counseling/psychotherapy and thus it is vital to control for.

Over one-half of the 38 men studied sometime during their psychotherapeutic contact experienced anxiety, but it did not increase over time. In the severe symptomatic phase (phase 3) anxiety correlated significantly with concerns such as work, housing, economy, or leisuretime. In the terminal disease phase (phase 4) HIV-related concerns, sexuality, and relationships triggered anxiety among the gay men.

Suicide

As with other life-threatening illness, such as cancer,[26] HIV has the potential of influencing suicidality. Although there is some evidence that people with HIV are at an increased risk of suicide compared to those without the infection,[27] Sherr[28] underscores the difficulties in gauging the prevalence of suicide due to methodological problems. Further, she points out that many researchers have focused only on death by suicide "rather than exploring the extreme mental health burden brought about by suicidal thoughts, attempts, completion and bereavement"[28] (p. 109).

Empirical research literature displays a diversified pattern with regard to suicidal risks among gay men with HIV. Some studies report an elevated risk for suicidal ideation, suicide attempts, and suicide in people with AIDS.[29,30] However, Beckett et al.[31] found in their review that people with HIV but without AIDS were more likely to exhibit suicidal ideation than those diagnosed with AIDS. Sherr et al. conclude that "a bimodal distribution of suicidal acts with peaks at or around diagnosis (of HIV) and again at the end stage of the illness"[32] was shown in a large collaborative study. Still other investigators have failed to find a correlation between suicide risk and people with AIDS[33,34] or men who are asymptomatic[16] or after HIV testing.[35] In a study on AIDS long-term survivors,[36] there were no attempted suicides after an AIDS diagnosis for individuals who had no prior suicidal history. Those two men who reported suicide attempts had done so prior to their AIDS diagnosis and in neither case was the attempt related to AIDS. None reported current suicidal ideation, although some considered it a future option should their condition became intolerable. In a case note audit study[28] the incidence of suicidal attempts was 21% and one-half of the sample was noted to have suicidal ideations. Those who had attempted suicide as well as those who expressed ideation were more likely to be HIV positive and well or diagnosed with AIDS.

Although the data are incongruent, there seems to be consensus among researchers that an earlier psychiatric history of depression and a history of attempted suicide are better predictors of current suicidal activity than an HIV diagnoses or diagnosis of HIV-related symptoms or diseases.[37–39] Various forms of substance use, grief, bereavement, and cumulative stressors also seem to correlate to suicide.[28,38,39]

In talking about "suicide" we suggest that it is necessary to make a distinction between suicide in the context of clinical depression and "acute" impulse-driven suicide on the one hand, and on the other hand philosophical suicide or "self-determined" or "accelerated" death.[40] The latter refers to a kind of contingency plan—killing oneself if medical conditions become unbearable. The possibility of choosing one's time of death may give the person a sense of personal control—to be in charge of death—and to sustain human dignity.

Over the years Dr. Schönnesson has worked with gay men with HIV, there is one man who committed suicide and another who made a serious suicide attempt. Tom wrote his self-determined death script. He left a letter explaining why he had decided to end his life. There were many reasons, but it was quite clear that Tom had considered his suicide carefully; a decision he regarded as "a good one," and he emphasized that suicide is a possibility for anyone. Larry, on the other hand, attempted suicide out of desperation but also as a way to tell his boyfriend, who was also HIV seropositive, that he did not have a "monopoly" on suffering. It was also a way to get control over the situation, because "my partner did his best to possess me but I did not want to be engulfed by him and therefore I had to disappear on my own account."

One half of the gay men discussed suicide issues in the course of their psychotherapeutic work. The theme was more salient in the asymptomatic and the severe symptomatic disease phases. Most of them talked about suicide in terms of self-determined death. But to others suicidal ideation may be frightening. Bob explains: "I'm afraid to lose control and to do something stupid like I do when I get my rage outbursts throwing things around me." About two years later Bob called the therapist (during that period of time they had had no psychotherapeutic contact). He told her that he had made a suicidal, however not serious, attempt. While the whole situation was strange and inexplicable to him he asked for some sessions to "sort things out." After three sessions Bob terminated (an intermittent termination) the counseling.

> Now I've got it all together and I can see that my suicidal attempt was a reaction to my body's deterioration. You know, it's tough to know that one is going to be blind pretty soon.

Those men who brought up suicidal issues were also focused on existential concerns and expressed a sense of hopelessness.

Mood Distress

Gay men living with HIV may also experience less severe, but still mentally painful, HIV-related reactions. They can be summarized under the heading of mood distress including global assessment of degree of distress as well as emotions such as anger, aloneness, resignation or hopelessness, helplessness, and despair. Clement et al.[17] note, however, that it is impossible to draw any conclusions with respect to associations between mood distress, HIV status group, and disease phases in that the methodologies of the studies are too heterogeneous. Longitudinal data indicate that gay men with HIV tend to have higher distress scores than their HIV-negative counterparts, but the difference does not increase over time.

Although a sense of hopelessness appears to be common among gay men with HIV, their scores are within the "mild hopelessness" range.[2,3,9] The quantitative analysis displayed that the vast majority of the gay men talked about feelings of hopelessness, but its intensity did not increase over time. We also found that the longer the man had known about his HIV diagnosis, the more hopelessness he experienced. At the end of the psychotherapeutic work—either self-terminated or by death—these feelings had decreased. It is highly plausible that this was at least partly a function of counseling and may be different in uncounseled men.

The vast majority of the gay men in Dr. Schönnesson's case load experienced feelings of exhaustion and/or resignation, despair, disappointment, violation, helplessness, and powerlessness. One-third and one-half of the men expressed anger and feelings of aloneness respectively. From a commonsense perspective it makes perfect sense that HIV may evoke all these moods. However, our data display a more complex picture, as is illustrated in Table 3.

First, all the moods except despair, exhaustion, or resignation were significantly related to HIV concerns. Second, some of these relationships were more

Table 3. Mood States over the Four HIV Disease Phases

The asymptomatic phase	The mild symptomatic phase	The severe symptomatic phase	The terminal phase
Anger	*Anger*	Anger	Anger
Helplessness	Helplessness	Helplessness	Helplessness
Powerlessness	Powerlessness	Powerlessness	Powerlessness
Disappointment	Disappointment	Disappointment	*Disappointment*
Violation	Violation	Violation	*Violation*
Aloneness	Aloneness	Aloneness	*Aloneness*

salient in some disease phases than in others (marked in italics in the table). Anger was induced by HIV concerns in the asymptomatic phase and by HIV-related symptoms in the mild symptomatic phase. Feelings of aloneness, disappointment, and violation and HIV concerns correlated significantly in the terminal phase.

Whereas there were no changes in the intensity of the above-mentioned moods over the disease phases, feelings of anger, disappointment, and violation, but also exhaustion/resignation decreased in the course of the psychotherapeutic counseling. Again, the counseling may have been the cause of this and constituted an artifact in the disease process.

Psychological distress also represents a risk factor of developing sexual symptoms, which in turn may reinforce perceived distress. Psychological distress may also be superimposed on sexual symptoms that are of a medical character.

The degree of mood distress can also be reinforced by HIV-related physical symptoms[7,9,16,22,25,41,42] and psychosocial factors such as low self-esteem,[42,44–46] AIDS-stress,[47] internalized anti-gay attitudes,[43,48–50] and self-blame for contracting the HIV-infection.[20,51,52] In their study, Wagner et al.[50] found that stronger internalized anti-gay attitudes at baseline, specifically among those men who were asymptomatic, predicted higher levels of distress two years later. No association between disease phases and internalized anti-gay attitudes was found. Both internalized anti-homosexual attitudes and self-blame carry with them elements of shame and/or guilt. Among the Swedish gay men, shame and guilt were significantly associated with sexuality and existential concerns in the asymptomatic and the severe symptomatic phases respectively. It is notable that shame and guilt were less salient in the terminal phase.

Given the uncertainty of life expectancy and disease progression one would expect gay men to report degrees of worries and subjectively perceived vulnerability to developing AIDS. Taylor et al.[53] report that thoughts of developing AIDS were the most stressful AIDS-related event. In Nilsson Schönnesson's cross-sectional study[47] two AIDS stress patterns were identified: the depressive ruminative and anxious/helpless pattern. The vast majority of the men reported moderate levels on either of the patterns. These patterns were significantly associated with worries about developing AIDS and a higher perceived risk to develop AIDS than other gay men.

As said before, all the 38 gay men experienced and talked about their worries related to HIV. In addition, one-half of these gay men also experienced and talked about nonspecific worries and fear. In the quantitative analysis, we found that these unspecified worries significantly correlated with HIV concerns in the asymptomatic phase (phase 1) and with HIV-related symptoms in the mild symptomatic phase (phase 2). It is highly plausible that experienced worries in the asymptomatic phase are related to uncertainty of disease progression and its potential consequences. Because symptoms start to develop in the mild symptomatic phase, it is understandable that the men expressed their physical worries during this second phase.

A closely linked issue is the impact of HIV/AIDS concerns on psychological functioning. Studies[24,54] indicate that AIDS concerns intrude on work, social relations, and mood status and are associated with pessimism as to HIV disease progression. Another study[47] implies that depressive and anxious AIDS stress patterns displayed HIV-related feelings of despair, hopelessness, powerlessness, and depressiveness as well as dissatisfaction with health and sexual life. Whereas general anxiety and depression do not seem to increase over time, AIDS concerns do.[24]

The quantitative analysis of the psychotherapeutic notes displayed a similar pattern. There was a decrease in *frequency* of men talking about HIV, but in those who did, there was an increased *intensity* in talking about HIV concerns over the disease phases. Anxiety and depression did not change over time. Joseph et al.[24] argue that it appears as though gay men with HIV "compartmentalize" their AIDS concerns and thus do not have an impact on their overall psychological functioning.

Grief

Gay men with HIV are confronted with separation, grief, and mourning processes in that HIV-related threats are ultimately related to potential losses. As was discussed in Chapter 4, not only are gay men faced with distress related to their own health but also to sickness and death of those around them. American authors[55,56] talk about "disenfranchised grief" among gay men. "That is, given society's homophobia, men who lose friends and loved ones to AIDS do not have adequate opportunity to mourn their deaths."[56]

Somewhat surprisingly, only a minority of the Swedish gay men (18%) expressed grief and loss. One obvious question is whether these men expressed their grief and mourning by using other words. It could for example be argued that grief might turn into a sense of hopelessness, meaninglessness, or emptiness (a kind of resignation). Data showed a significant correlation between grief and resignation and thus it could be argued that these men rather spoke in terms of resignation than grief (over two-thirds of the men expressed resignation). However, this association vanished when disease phases were controlled for, which might be explained by the relatively small sample.

Considering the grief scenario a relevant question is what the consequence of multiple bereavement is. Maasen[57] notes that depression, survival guilt, and shame of being gay are common symptoms of pervasive loss. He further argues that as the trauma of loss is ongoing it gets integrated in the personality, "which means it [loss] becomes chronic and will complicate the mourning process"[57] (p. 58). The effect of experiencing multiple losses on a variety of psychological symptoms in a sample of gay men with and without HIV over one year was studied by Gluboski et al.[58] Their findings indicate that experiencing two or more losses in the year prior to the first interview was associated with higher levels of distress in follow-up assessment over one year. Gay men with HIV, in comparison to their negative counterparts, displayed higher levels of distress on all measures, except for intrusive and avoidant thoughts and images. Results from a New York study[59] indicate that the types of distress most reactive to AIDS-related loss were intrusive and avoidant thoughts and emotions about AIDS (often associated with post-traumatic stress disorder), depression, hopelessness, helplessness—symptoms associated with being demoralized—and sleep problems. These symptoms increased directly with the number of bereavements. A German study[56] among gay men living with HIV showed that losing a partner or close friend to AIDS, denying the effects that AIDS has on one's life, and experiencing a general sense of demoralization explained 77% of the variance in post-traumatic stress disorder. Having HIV also correlated with post-traumatic stress disorder but did not contribute significantly to the regression model. As Wright emphasizes, "It is an indication that HIV is strongly correlated with variables entered into the equation as well as with other predictors of stress"[56] (p. 4).

Couple and Psychological Functioning

All the studies presented above are focused on the individual. Despite the fact that many gay men with HIV are committed to intimate relationships, very few studies pay attention to the couple and its degree of psychological distress. In a male couple study[60] of serodiscordant status relationships, the investigators found elevated levels of self-reported depression, anxiety, hostility, hopelessness, and distress in both members of the couple. This indicates that both the man with HIV as well as the HIV-seronegative partner are affected by HIV. The strongest predictors of distress were poor communication and avoidance, lack of social support from partner and community, lack of sexual and general relationship satisfaction, and difficulty in finding meaning in an uncertain future.

THE INFLUENCE OF PSYCHOLOGICAL AND SOCIAL MEDIATORS ON PSYCHOLOGICAL FUNCTIONING

As stated above, gay men with HIV are exposed to both chronically stressful situations (HIV-infection as such) as well as stressful events (e.g., HIV-related threats and psychological issues). They may respond to their HIV disease and related threats and stressors with a range of distress symptoms. In other words, people differ in terms of vulnerability[61] or have unequal success when dealing with the same hardships. How can we account for these individual differences?

The cognitive theory on stress and coping[62] emphasizes that the relationship between stressful situations and psychological distress symptoms is mediated by situational appraisals of control and coping. Dohrenwend[1] also focuses, in her model of life stress process, on the central role of mediating factors in the influence that stressors may ultimately have on individual psychological well-being. "Stress reaction interacts with situational [social support] and psychological mediators [self-esteem, coping, and mastery] to produce any of three general outcomes"[1] (p. 5). Possible outcomes are not only psychological distress, but also personal growth or a status quo (no substantial psychological change).

The hitherto most studied stress mediators within HIV-related psychosocial research are coping and social support. But there are also other psychological stress mediators that play a role in the process, such as subjective attribution theories to HIV and subjective perception of disease control. However, these are not nearly as well studied as coping and social support. Little is known about the relative importance of any of the stress mediators as well as the impact of personality characteristics and the way they interact in reducing mood distress. Our knowledge is also sparse as to whether stress mediators play different roles depending on disease phases. Further, there is a void in our understanding about whether the mediating factors (or the mediating profile) may differ depending on the type of threat or stressor in focus.

Coping

Coping is assumed to play a major role in any stress process and many (non-HIV related) studies have been conducted to understand "the relationship of particular sorts of coping strategies to outcomes in the stress process"[63] (p. 13). They also show that different situations call forth different kinds of coping.

Coping is commonly used interchangeably with concepts such as mastery, defense, and adaptation,[64] and it has acquired a range of meanings. Pearlin and Schooler refer to coping as "any response to external life-strains that serves to prevent, avoid, or control emotional distress"[65] (p. 3). Maybe the most well-known definition is the one by Lazarus and Folkman: "[coping refers to] constantly changing cognitive and behavioral efforts to manage specific external and/or internal demands that are appraised as taxing or exceeding the resources of the person"[62] (p. 141). In Lazarus and Folkman's perspective, adaptation to a stressful situation/event is a dynamic process. It is formed by cognitive appraisals of the situation/event in terms of harm/loss, threat and/or challenge, their suffused emotional response, and by behaviors and thoughts related to coping with the situation/event. Coping has two major functions: to manage or alter the problem that is causing distress (problem-focused coping) and to regulate emotional responses to the problem (emotion-focused coping).[66]

Similar to non-HIV studies, research on the impact of coping on psychological distress within the HIV realm indicates that the use of "negative" coping styles, such as wishful thinking, avoidance, isolation, and fatalism, is associated with increased distress and diminished well-being.[42–46,49,67–70] Conversely, problem solving, positive reappraisal, and information seeking are related to decreased psychological distress.[42–46]

We suggest that a given coping strategy or a coping style could not automatically be assessed as adaptive or maladaptive. (Here we use the term *strategy* to refer to a conscious choice of a coping mechanism, while "style" refers to a less conscious mechanism based on the person's personality.) For example, an avoidant coping style/strategy may under certain conditions be an adaptive way to "dose" painful emotions and experiences, thus protecting the individual from being overwhelmed by these feelings. But the same style given other conditions may end up being maladaptive. We also have to bear in mind that a given coping strategy/style may have different psychological functions depending on which personality it is embedded in. For example, a pro-active coping strategy/style may function as a defensive compensation for a fragile self-esteem, but it could also be a reflection of internal and well-grounded resources.

Social Support

The concept of social support is an "omnibus term" relating to different aspects of social relationships. It includes: (1) the network structure or social interactions, (2) emotional, psychological, tangible or informational support, and (3) the perceived quality or adequacy of this support.[71] There seems to be consensus among researchers[72] that access to social support and perceptions of feeling supported are important buffers (referred to as the buffering model of social support[73]) to the negative psychological consequences of stressful experiences. When it comes to life-threatening diseases, it is highly likely that social support needs and type of support may vary over the course of the disease.

Social support and HIV has been studied in relation to its impact on physical health but in particular psychological functioning. In her review, Green concludes that based on existing findings it is unclear

> whether good social support promotes longevity or whether those who progress more quickly find support diminishing as a result of reduced social interaction or friends' fearful avoidance of them.[71] (p. 97)

Although some studies have found a relationship between certain aspects of social support and self-reported physical health, Green emphasizes that as of yet, no significant correlation has been found between objective measures of health status and social support.

Empirical data on the impact of satisfaction with, or perceived availability of, social support on psychological functioning appears to be consistent. Several studies[16,43,45,46,48,71,74] conclude that social support has proved to reduce psychological distress among gay men living with HIV. In Hays et al.'s[75] study data showed that those gay men who were satisfied with the social support they received were less likely to show current depression or increased depression one year later. Similar results have been found among people with cancer; the amount of social support at time of diagnosis is positively linked to psychological well-being up to two years later and even with patients' length of life.[76] Presentations at the eleventh international AIDS conference in Vancouver in 1996 clearly demonstrated the positive value of perceived emotional support, contact with friends and family, community-based supportive services, and the negative value of interpersonal conflict.[77] Further, data imply that gay men perceive partners and close friends as more supportive and helpful than family members in dealing with HIV infection.[43,55,71,74,78]

In contrast, Fleishman and Fogel's[42] measure of the number of close friends and relatives and perceived tangible support were not strongly related to support seeking. Based on their findings, Fleishman and Fogel argue that seeking support may be a response to distress; that is, when distress reaches unacceptable levels the individual seeks support. But it would appear as though the individual's attempt to mobilize his potential social network may not be successful. "These findings point to the importance of distinguishing support seeking from receipt of support"[42] (p. 164).

Just as social interactions can be of support, they can also be a source of stress, as being unhelpful or negative. Ingram et al.[79] point out that negative interactions may have important adverse consequences on psychological functioning and may be particularly salient for people with HIV, given the stigma attached to the disease. Within such a perspective it is, as Ingram et al. emphasize, surprising that so little attention has been paid to the nature of and effects of negative social interactions. In their study, Ingram et al. developed a measure to assess HIV-related unsupportive or upsetting social interactions. They could identify four types of unsupportive responses that people with HIV might receive from others: insensitivity, disconnecting, forced optimism, and blaming. Their findings suggest that unsupportive social interactions and social support are relatively independent constructs. Moreover, data revealed that persons who reported more HIV-related unsupportive social interactions also reported being more depressed. Unsupportive social interactions predicted a significant amount of variance in depression, beyond the variance accounted for by physical functioning and positive social support. Ingram et al. conclude:

> Consistent with the findings of Siegel et al. (1994, 1997) our results highlight the importance of assessing positive social support and negative social interactions separately, and suggest that these variables make independent contributions to well-being among people with HIV.[79]

As pointed out in Chapter 4, the social network of gay men appears to shrink at the time of the HIV notification. It is, however, unclear whether this change in the network is a consequence of withdrawal by other people or whether the individual avoids relations because of depressiveness, low self-esteem, or fear of being abandoned. Many of the men with HIV who were consulted by Dr. Schönnesson reported that they had reduced their social network very consciously. Tom's remark is typical:

> I have become much more picky and critical when it comes to friends and acquaintances. I very much prefer to have a few, real close friends whom I can rely on than a whole bunch of people.

But what is it about social support that is beneficial? Various researchers[80,81] have made attempts to distinguish between various functions of social support (emotional, instrumental, material, informational) in order to explicate how and when support is effective. The emotional-sustaining types of help appear to be the most desirable by people with HIV,[71] although they are not significantly correlated to physical health or psychological well-being. Hays et al.,[41] on the other hand, found that (HIV/AIDS-related) informational support was especially critical in buffering depression for men experiencing HIV-related symptoms. It could be speculated that informational support is important and stress reducing in that it contributes to a sense of control and predictability over one's situation.[41] Thoits[82] argues that coping and social support have several functions in common, and, therefore, social support can be conceptualized as coping assistance. Some studies[45,46] show that active-behavioral coping is related to higher levels of perceived social support and avoidance coping to less social support. These findings could be understood in terms of those who cope in an "adaptive" way with a crisis are more likely to be liked and supported by others. On the other hand, the "avoidant copers" who are in the greatest need of social support are the least likely to receive it.[45]

However, as Janoff-Bulman[83] concludes, the functional perspective of social support does not provide any understanding of the special role of other people after a traumatic life event. But this can be understood when we consider, as is to be discussed in Chapter 9, that following an overwhelming event such as the HIV diagnosis, the individual is involved in a reconstructing process of his self and his assumptive world. In this process persons play a crucial role just as they did in the child's development of his self and his identities. We need others to become someone, a person, to know who we are, as captured in sociologist Charles Cooley's (1902, cf. in Janoff-Bulman[83]) phrase "the looking-glass self" or in Kohut's words, the mirroring function of others.[84]

Subjective HIV Attribution Theories and Subjective Perception of Disease Control

Subjective attribution theories to HIV (further discussed in Chapter 7) refer to the individual's psychological explanation(s) of HIV infection by means of its attribution to the self, some other person, the environment, or chance.[52]

The mediator of subjective perception of disease control implies different subjective theories as to whether the HIV infection can be controlled either by the individual himself (internal locus of control), by others (external locus of control), or by chance. A sense of control is important as a means to live with the uncertainties of the HIV infection. Weitz[85] states, that when there is no or a low degree of sense of control it may lead to experiences of stress and depression. A vast, non-HIV, empirical literature demonstrates that when people de facto can or believe they have control over a difficult situation they will adapt better to it.[86,87] Moulton et al.[88] found in their study that those gay men with HIV who were convinced they could influence their health by means of changes in style of living also displayed a lower degree of psychological distress. Another study[3] among gay men with HIV showed that the higher sense of health control they perceived the more resilient they were, whereas those men who experienced external control were more likely to experience helplessness as to future. In Nilsson Schönnesson's[47] study data showed a significant correlation between a positive self-image and a strong sense of internal control over the HIV infection. Those men who viewed themselves as being in control of the disease also rated their risk of developing AIDS as minimal.

QUALITY OF LIFE

The concept of quality of life has attracted the attention of numerous researchers particularly within the health care context. According to Brown, Renwick, and Nagler,[89] the interest in quality of life stems from trends toward greater appreciation of the personal needs and wishes of individuals within the health and social services. Although the concept has been and is used frequently there is no exact definition or thorough conceptualization of quality of life. It is generally described in terms of positive subjective judgments such as happiness, satisfaction, well-being, and a subjective feeling of experiencing a good life. Empirical research indicates that all of these concepts have been used inconsistently and that many have been used interchangeably.[89] As quality of life is assumed to be a broader concept than the others, it could be argued that quality of life may subsume concepts such as happiness and life satisfaction. In a clinical setting, according to Franchi and Wenzel, the definition of quality of life is "limited to those aspects of life directly affected by the heath state ... and is often referred to as health-related quality of life"[90] (p. 20).

Traditionally quality of life has been related to health status in that health is considered to be one of the most important contributing factors to overall quality of life.[91] But quality of life is also thought of as a determinant of overall health. Terms such as functional status or health status are commonly used as synonyms for quality of life in spite of the fact that they were developed as measures of function and health. This health-related approach to "quality of life" does not acknowledge the individual's perception but relies on the researcher's assessment of quality of life.

Another approach to quality of life is characterized by the focus on the individual's subjective evaluation of well-being independent of health status. Just as severe disease does not necessarily cause illness (poor subjective health), studies show that despite a severe disease people are able to maintain a feeling of well-being and satisfaction with life. One plausible explanation of the retention of quality of life during severe disease may be that the individual attributes meaning to suffering and in that way is able to integrate painful events into his life.

Generally speaking quality of life is viewed as being socially constructed and multidimensional. There can be no absolute value of quality of life as there are many different cultural values and expectations on what constitutes quality of life, and cultural values may vary from group to group. Ross and Ryan[92] take as an example the male gay culture. Since sexuality has such a central place in the definition of the gay identity and in the construction of the HIV disease, sexuality is a central component of quality of life definitions. Within this context it is interesting to note that in Nilsson Schönnesson's study on quality of life[93] among gay men with HIV, sexuality (in terms of "having sex") was not included as an aspect of their subjective perception of quality of life. On the other hand, the importance of intimacy and love were emphasized by many of the men. At least among these men, intimacy appears to be higher valued than having sex with respect to quality of life. On the other hand, we suggest that because of the Swedish Communicable Disease Act, the men might be more hesitant and reluctant to acknowledge that having sex is important to them. From that perspective, intimacy and love are more legitimate aspects of quality of life.

The multidimensional character of quality of life is reflected in the variety of aspects or domains of life that are included in instruments measuring quality of life. The vast majority of the traditional constructed scales focused on measuring the impact of a given disease on physical functioning and to a lesser extent psychological well-being. Current researchers underscore the importance of including not only physical but also psychological, social, and cognitive functions as well as intimacy or sexual functioning, community, and spiritual domains. We would also suggest that as HIV evokes existential concerns, they ought to be acknowledged when assessing quality of life. But it is not clear whether the existential dimension should be seen as a subdomain of quality of life or as a separate variable interacting with it. Only further empirical research will be able to provide us with an answer.

HIV-treatment advances and their expanding repertoire and increased life expectancy have contributed to a growing concern about the quality of life among people living with HIV. We find this "upswing" in interest as notable, as quality of life, from our standpoint, should always be at focus regardless of disease phase, treatment options, or longevity. However, empirical research is still sparse and most of it is so far related to quality of life incorporated as an outcome measure in clinical trials for medication (see review by Franchi and Wenzel[90]). Several generic instruments have been used (e.g., quality of well-being[94]) but also generic instruments that are adapted to people with HIV (e.g., various forms from the Medical Outcomes Study[95]). Another instrument is the Functional Assessment of Human Immunodeficiency (FAHI)[96] virus infection, which was originally developed for people with cancer. Yet, these and other quality of life analytical instruments are criticized. One criticism is that they have been developed with very little input from people with HIV.[97] To quote Holmes and Shea, "[the instruments"] appear to have been driven mostly by investigators' beliefs about quality of life in HIV infection and not to have included much or any input from HIV seropositive individuals[97] (p. 430). Further, scales being used are usually based on lifestyles and are concerned more typically with heterosexual, married, and older cancer patients. Usually they do not have an index score on quality of life.

HIV-specific measures developed through input of individuals with HIV are rare, although it is most likely that such a procedure will result in a relevant instrument including dimensions that are of concern to people with HIV. However, we are aware of two exceptions. Holmes and Shea[97] have developed the HIV/AIDS-targeted Quality of Life (HAT-QoL) instrument. It is a five dimension quality of life instrument including overall function, disclosure worries, health worries, financial worries, and life satisfaction. The second instrument, The Fanning Quality of Life[98] scale, is a 37-item questionnaire. It asks the respondent to rate on a seven-point Likert scale the degree to which different aspects of his or her life (for example social life, spiritual beliefs) have been affected by HIV and how positive or negative the effect has been.

A common assumption by laypeople is that people with HIV/AIDS experience an impoverished quality of life. In addition, researchers tend to assign to their respondents who are sick a lower quality of life than the people themselves do.[74] Quality of life may even be increased when people get seriously ill with their HIV infection.[22,99] In their review of existing studies on health-related quality of life, Franchi and Wenzel conclude that "health-related quality of life scores do not always correlate with disease stage or health indices and that symptoms have a significant impact on HRQL [health-related quality of life]"[90] (p. 20). Whereas Cleary et al.[100] found that both physical health status and psychological functioning status correlated with and predicted life satisfaction, other studies[2,19] suggest that degree of physical impairment is not related to life satisfaction. Holmes et al.[101] studied the effect of Axis I psychiatric disorders on psychological well-being and quality of life. Their findings indicate that the presence of Axis I psychiatric disorders in the previous six months is associated with diminished scores in multiple areas of functioning and well-being, independent of HIV-related disease progression. Holmes et al. conclude that Axis 1 disorders therefore appear to impact quality of life. It also appears to be a negative relationship between clinical depression and quality of life.[94,102] Rubin et al.[102] reported that those who developed depressive symptoms over a six-month period showed a decline in their quality of well-being scores.

Coping and social support may influence quality of life, just as does psychological functioning. Still, we know little about the relationship between various types of social support, coping styles/strategies, and domains of quality of life as well as their relationship to disease and illness. Renwich and Friedland[103] conducted a study on coping, social support, and quality of life in persons with HIV. Because of the multidimensional character of quality of life three different types of measurements were used; behavioral aspects of quality of life (e.g., job satisfaction, personal growth), health-related quality of life (different aspects of life that have been affected by HIV), and life satisfaction. The participants scored lower on overall quality of life, physical well-being, material well-being, vacation behavior, and partner relationship than the norm groups. Findings indicate that health status is not a useful indicator for assessment of quality of life. Further, data showed that different types of social support and coping strategies influenced different aspects of quality of life. Problem-oriented coping, lack of denial, and emotional social support influenced behavioral dimensions of quality of life. Emotional social support in combination with the absence of practical support and perception-oriented coping (e.g., positive reappraisal of one's situation) positively affected health-related quality of life. The researchers conclude:

> one major implication of the study for assessment and intervention was that different combinations of coping strategies and social supports are potentially valuable for improving different aspects of quality of life.[103] (p. 188)

We find empirical knowledge being minimal as to (1) the ways people with HIV themselves define the concept of quality of life; (2) the types of potential stressors (for example, how stressful combination therapy may be perceived) and their impact on quality of life; (3) psychological, existential, and social mediators that may exacerbate or moderate the impact of stressors on quality of life, and (4) to what extent definitions, stressors, and mediators differ depending on disease stage and whether the individual is on treatment regimens. We also have to discuss and study to what extent there might exist some basic components of quality of life that are more or less common to most people, but where we might ascribe different meanings or importance to these components depending upon our health status. The importance might also change over time. We also raise the question whether it might be more correct to talk about quality of life profiles rather than a single measure of degree of quality of life.

SUMMARY

Empirical and clinical data show that gay men with HIV react to the HIV disease in a variety of ways, from psychiatric disorders to transient mood distress. Although clinical depression has received much attention, data are still inconclusive with respect to prevalence of depression and whether rates increase with progression. A similar conclusion can be drawn as to suicide. However, empirical and clinical data indicate that HIV concerns increase over disease phases. Further, clinical data displayed that HIV concerns appeared to trigger anger in the asymptomatic and mild symptomatic phases, whereas aloneness, disappointment, and violation were triggered in the terminal phase. Unspecific worries, as experienced by those gay men, related to HIV concerns in the asymptomatic phase and to HIV-related symptoms in the mild symptomatic phase. Empirical research clearly implies that experiencing multiple loss and bereavement has a negative impact on psychological well-being. Coping and social support are up until the present the most studied stress mediators. Empirical data are congruent in that avoidant coping is related to increased distress, and social support reduces distress. Those men who perceive themselves to be in control of their HIV infection are less distressed and more resilient. Finally, studies show that health-related quality of life does not always correlate with disease phase or health indices. On the contrary, quality of life may even increase when people get seriously ill with their HIV infection.

REFERENCES

1. Dohrenwend B. Social stress and community psychology. *American Journal of Community Psychology* 1978; 6(1):1–14.
2. Rabkin J, Remien RH, Katoff L, *et al.* Resilience in adversity among long-term survivors with AIDS. *Hospital Community Psychiatry* 1993; 44:162–167.
3. Rabkin J, Williams J, Neugebauer R, *et al.* Maintenance of hope in HIV-spectrum of homosexual men. *American Journal of Psychiatry* 1990; 147(10):1322–1327.
4. Thompson SC, Nanni C, Levine A. The stressors and stress of being HIV-positive. *AIDS Care* 1996; 9(1):5–14.
5. Atkinson JH, Grant I, Bennedy CJ, *et al.* Prevalence of psychiatric disorders among men infected with human immunodeficiency virus. *Archives of General Psychiatry* 1988; 45:859–864.
6. Williams J, Rabkin J, Remien RH, *et al.* Multidisciplinary baseline assessment of homosexual men with and without human immunodeficiency virus infection. *Archives of General Psychiatry* 1991; 48:124–130.
7. Perry SW, Jacobsberg LB, Card C, *et al.* Severity of psychiatric symptoms after HIV testing. *American Journal of Psychiatry* 1993; 150:775–779.
8. Perkins DO, Stern R, Golden R. Mood disorders in HIV infection: prevalence and risk factors in nonepicenter of the AIDS epidemic. *American Journal of Psychiatry* 1994; 151:223–236.
9. Rabkin J, Ferrando SJ, Jacobsberg LB, *et al.* Prevalence of Axis I in an AIDS cohort; a cross-sectional, controlled study. *Comprehensive Psychiatry* 1997; 38(3):146–154.
10. McDaniel JS, Musselman DI, Porter MR, *et al.* Depression in patients with cancer: diagnosis, biology, and treatment. *Archives of General Psychiatry* 1995; 52:89–99.
11. Atkinson JH, Grant I. Natural history of neuropsychiatric manifestations of HIV disease. *Psychiatric Clinics of North America* 1994; 17(1):17–33.
12. Dilley JW, Ochitill HN, Perl M, *et al.* Findings in psychiatric consultations with patients with acquired immune deficiency syndrome. *American Journal of Psychiatry* 1985; 142:82–86.
13. Nichols S. Psychological reactions of persons with AIDS. *Annals of Internal Medicine* 1985; 103:765–767.

14. Tross S, Hirsch D, Rabkin, J, *et al.* Determinants of current psychiatric disorder in AIDS spectrum patients. Proceedings of the 3rd International Conference on AIDS, Washington D.C.; 1987.
15. Perdices M, Dunbar N, Grunseit A, *et al.* Anxiety, depression, and HIV-related symptomatology across the spectrum of HIV disease. *Australian New Zealand Journal of Psychiatry* 1992; 26: 560–566.
16. Ostrow DG, Monjan A, Joseph JG, *et al.* HIV-related symptoms and psychological functioning in a cohort of homosexual men. *American Journal of Psychiatry* 1989; 146:737–742.
17. Clement U, Gramatikov L, Laszig P, *et al. Förderschewerpunkt AIDS, Bereich Sozialwissenschaften des BMFT/BMBT. Methodische integration von empirischen Studien zur Lebensqualität, psychischen Verarbeitung und sexuellen Verhalten HIV-Infizierter. Absclussbericht.* Psychosomatische Klinik, Universität Heidelberg; 1997.
18. Bayer R. Clinical progress and the future of HIV exceptionalism, Paper presented at the 2nd European conference on the methods and results of social and behavioral research on AIDS, Paris January 12–15; 1998.
19. Chuang HT, Devins GM, Hunsley J, *et al.* Psychosocial distress and well-being among gay and bisexual men with immunodeficiency virus infection. *American Journal of Psychiatry* 1989; 146:876–880.
20. Moulton JM, Stempel RR, Bacchetti P, *et al.* Results of one year longitudinal study of HIV antibody test notification from the San Francisco General Hospital cohort. *Journal of Acquired Immune Deficiency Syndromes* 1991; 4:787–794.
21. Franke GH. *Die psychosoziale Situation von HIV-Positiven.* Berlin: Ergebnisse sozialwissenschaftlicher Aids-Forschung 5. edition sigma; 1990.
22. Rabkin J, Williams JB, Remien RH, *et al.* Depression, distress, lymphocyte subsets, and human immunodeficiency virus symptoms on ten occasions in HIV-positive homosexual men. *Archives of General Psychiatry* 1991; 48:111–119.
23. Rabkin J, Goetz RR, Remien RH, *et al.* Stability of mood despite HIV illness progression in a group of homosexual men. *American Journal of Psychiatry* 154(2):231–238.
24. Joseph JG, Caumartin S, Tal M, *et al.* Psychological functioning in a cohort of gay men at risk for AIDS. A three-year descriptive study. *Journal of Nervous and Mental Disease* 1990; 178: 607–615.
25. Lyketsos CG, Hoover DR, Guccione M, *et al.* Depressive symptoms as predictors of medical outcomes in HIV infection: Multicenter AIDS cohort study. *JAMA* 1993; 270:2563–2567.
26. Allebeck P, Bolund C. Suicides and suicide attempts in cancer patients. *Psychological Medicine* 1991; 21:976–984.
27. Catalan J, Pugh K. Suicidal behavior and HIV infection—is there a link? *AIDS Care* 1995; 7:S117–S121.
28. Sherr L. Suicide and AIDS: lessons from a case note audit in London. *AIDS Care* 1995; 7:S109–S116.
29. Halstead S, Riccio M, Harlow P, *et al.* Psychosis associated with HIV infection. *British Journal of Psychiatry* 1988; 153:618–623.
30. Marzuk P, Tierney H, Tardiff K, *et al.* Increased risk of suicide in persons with AIDS. *Journal of the American Medical Association* 1988; 259:1333–1337.
31. Beckett A, Shenson D, *et al.* Suicide risk in patients with human immunodeficiency virus infection and AIDS. *Harvard Review of Psychiatry* 1993; 1:27–35.
32. Sherr L, Campbell J, Neil L, *et al.* Suicide and AIDS—A report of the European initiative. Oral presentation, abstract WeD.242 at the 11th International Conference on AIDS, Vancouver, Canada; 1996.
33. McKegney FP, O'Dowd MA. Suicidality and HIV status. *American Journal of Psychiatry* 1992; 149:396–398.
34. O'Dowd MA, McKegney FP. AIDS patients compared with others seen in psychiatric consultation. *General Hospital Psychiatry* 1990; 12:50–55.

35. Perry SW, Jacobsberg LB, Fishman B. Suicidal ideation and HIV testing. *Journal of the American Medical Association* 1990; 85:40–43.
36. Rabkin J, Remien RH, Katoff L, *et al.* Suicidality in AIDS long-term survivors: What is the evidence? *AIDS Care* 1993; 5(3):393–403.
37. Gala C, Pergami A, Catalan J, *et al.* Risk of deliberate self harm and factors associated with suicidal behavior among asymptomatic individuals with HIV. *Acta Psychiatrica Scandinavica* 1992; 86:70–75.
38. Gorman M, Wiley J, Winkelstein W, *et al.* Risk factors of suicide: Depression, alcohol, drug use, grief and bereavement. PoD 5471. 8th International Conference on AIDS, Amsterdam, Holland; 1992.
39. Schneider SG, Taylor SE, Hammen C, *et al.* Factors influencing suicide intent in gay and bisexual suicide ideators: differing models for men with and without human immunodeficiency virus. *Journal of Personality and Social Psychology* 1991; 6:776-788.
40. Rabkin J, Remien RH, Wilson C. *Good Doctors, Good Patients. Partners in HIV Treatment.* New York: NCM Publisher; 1994.
41. Hays RB, Turner H, Coates TJ. Social support, AIDS-related symptoms, and depression among gay men. *Journal of Consulting and Clinical Psychology* 1992; 60:463–469.
42. Fleishman JA, Fogel B. Coping and depressive symptoms among people with AIDS. *Health Psychology* 1994; 13(2):156–169.
43. Nicholson WD, Long BC. Self-esteem, social support, internalized homophobia, and coping strategies of HIV+ gay men. *Journal of Consulting and Clinical Psychology* 1990; 58:873–876.
44. Kurdek LA, Siesky G. The nature and correlates of psychological adjustment in gay men with AIDS-related conditions. *Journal of Applied Social Psychology* 1990; 20:846–860.
45. Namir S, Wolcott D, Fawsey FI, *et al.* Implications of different strategies for coping with AIDS. In: Temoshok L, Baum A, eds. *Psychosocial Perspectives on AIDS. Etiology, Prevention, and Treatment.* Hillsdale, N.J.: Lawrence Erlbaum; 1990; 173–190.
46. Wolf TM, Balson PM, Morse EV, *et al.* Relationship of coping style to affective state and perceived social support in asymptomatic and symptomatic HIV-infected persons: Implications for clinical management. *Journal of Clinical Psychology* 1991; 52:171–173.
47. Nilsson Schönnesson L. HIV infection: Trauma, psychic metabolism, and psychological wellbeing. A study of 29 gay HIV-positive men. Unpublished report (in Swedish). Stockholm: 1993.
48. Wolcott DL, Namir S, Fawzy FI, *et al.* Illness concerns, attitudes toward homosexuality, and social support in gay men with AIDS. *General Hospital Psychiatry* 1986; 8:395–403.
49. Weimer E, Clement U, Nilsson-Schönnesson L. Depressive Reaktionen und psychische Verarbeitung bei HIV-positiven homosexuellen Männern. *Psychotherapie Psychosomatik Medizinische Psychologie* 1991; 41:107–114
50. Wagner G, Brondolo E, Rabkin J. Internalized homophobia in a sample of HIV+ gay men, and its relationship to psychological distress, coping, and illness progression. *Journal of Homosexuality* 1996; 32(2):91–106.
51. Simeone A, Hermand D. Subjective health state and perceived social support in HIV infection. Poster PO97 presented at the AIDS' Impact—Biopsychosocial Aspects of HIV infection, 2nd International Conference, Brighton, England; 1994.
52. Clement U, Nilsson Schönnesson L. Subjective HIV attribution theories, coping, and psychological functioning among homosexual men with HIV. *AIDS Care* 1998; 10(3)355–366.
53. Taylor SE, Kemeny ME, Aspinwall LG, *et al.* Optimism, coping, psychological distress, and high-risk sexual behavior among men at risk for acquired immunodeficiency syndrome (AIDS). *Journal of Personality and Social Psychology* 1992; 63(3):460–473.
54. Hart CB, Taylor SE, Kemeny ME, *et al.* Positive and negative changes in response to the threat of AIDS: Psychological adjustment as a function of severity of threat and life domain. In: Program and abstracts: 6th International Conference on AIDS, San Francisco: Abstract S.B.371; 1990.

55. Hays RB, Chauncey S, Tobey LA. The social support networks of gay men with AIDS. *Journal of Community Psychology*. 1990; 18(4):374–385.
56. Wright, M. AIDS survivor syndrome and being HIV positive. Paper presented at the 2nd European conferece on the methods and results of social and behavioral research on AIDS, Paris, France, January 12–15, 1998.
57. Maasen T. Counseling gay men with multiple loss and survival problems: The bereavement group as a transitional object. *AIDS Care* 1998; 10(1):S57–S63.
58. Gluboski VI, Fishman B, Perry SW. The impact of multiple bereavement in a gay male sample. *AIDS Education and Prevention* 1997; 9(6):521–531.
59. Martin JL. Psychological consequences of AIDS-related bereavement among gay men. *Journal of Consulting and Clinical Psychology* 1988; 56(6):856–862.
60. Remien RH, Wagner G, Carballo-Dieguez A, *et al.* Psychological distress in male couples of mixed HIV status. Paper presented at the American Psychological Association Annual Meeting, August 9, 1996.
61. Kessler RC. A strategy for studying differential vulnerability to the psychological consequences of stress. *Journal of Health and Social Behavior* 1979; 20:100–108.
62. Lazarus RS, Folkman, S. *Stress, appraisal, and coping*. New York: Springer; 1984.
63. Wethington E., Kessler R. Situations and processes of coping. In: Eckenrode J, ed. *The Social Context of Coping*. New York: Plenum; 1991; 13–29.
64. White RW. Strategies of adaptation: An attempt at systematic description. In: Coehlo GV, Hamburg DA, Adams JE, eds. *Coping and Adaptation*. New York: Basic Books; 1974; 47–68.
65. Pearlin L, Schooler C. The structure of coping. *Journal of Health and Social Behavior* 1978; 19:2–21.
66. Folkman S, Lazarus RS. An analysis of coping in a middle-aged community sample. *Journal of Health and Social Behavior* 1980; 21:219–239.
67. Folkman S, Chesney M, Pollack I, *et al.* Stress, coping and depressive mood in human immunodeficiency virus-positive and negative gay men in San Francisco. *Journal of Nervous and Mental Disease* 1993; 181:409–416.
68. Clement U. *HIV-positiv. Psychische Verarbeitung, subjektive Infektionstheorien und psychosexuelle Konflikte HIV-Infizierter. Eine komparativ-kasuistische Studie*. Stuttgart: Ferdinand Enke Verlag; 1992.
69. Leserman J, Perkins DO, Evans DL. Coping with the threat of AIDS: the role of social support. *American Journal of Psychiatry* 1992; 149:1514–1520.
70. Antoni MH, Goodkin K, Goldstein D, *et al.* Coping responses to HIV-1 serostatus notification predict short-term affective distress and one-year follow-up immunological status in HIV-1 seronegative and seropositive gay men. *Psychosomatic Medicine* 1991; 53:244.
71. Green G. Editorial review: social support and HIV. *AIDS Care* 1993; 5:87–104.
72. Eckenrode J, ed. *The Social Context of Coping*. New York: Plenum; 1991.
73. Cohen S, Wills TA. Stress, social support, and the buffering hypothesis. *Psychological Bulletin* 1985; 98:310–357.
74. Friedland L, Renwick R, McColl M. Coping and social support as determinants of quality of life in HIV/AIDS. *AIDS Care* 1996; 8(1):15–32.
75. Hays RB, Turner H, Coates T. Social support, AIDS-related symptoms, and depression among gay men. *Journal of Consulting and Clinical Psychology* 1992; 60(3):463–469.
76. Dunkel-Schetter CA. Social support and cancer: Findings based on patient interviews and their implications. *Journal of Social Issues* 1984; 40:77–98.
77. Remien RH. Psychological distress and support. *Focus* 1996; 11(11):1–4.
78. Folkman S, Chesney M, Christopher-Richards A. Stress and coping in caregiving partners of men with AIDS. *Psychiatric Clinics of North America* 1994; 1:35–53.
79. Ingram K, Jones DA, Fass R, *et al.* Social support and unsupportive social interactions: Their association with depression among people living with HIV. *AIDS Care*, in press; 1998.

80. Cohen S, Wills TA. Stress, social support, and the buffering hypothesis. *Psychological Bulletin* 1985; 98:310–357.
81. Silver RL, Wortman CB. Coping with undesirable life events. In Garber J, Seligman MEP, eds. *Human Helplessness: Theory and Application.* New York: Academic Press; 1980.
82. Thoits PA. Social support as coping assistance. *Journal of Consulting and Clinical Psychology* 1985; 54:416–423.
83. Janoff-Bulman R. *Shattered assumptions. Towards a new psychology of trauma.* New York: Free Press; 1995.
84. Kohut H. *The Analysis of the Self.* New York: International Universities Press; 1971.
85. Weitz R. *Life with AIDS.* New Brunswick, N.J.: Rutgers University Press; 1992.
86. Thompson SC. Will it hurt less if I can control it? A complex answer to a simple question. *Psychological Bulletin* 1981; 90:89–101.
87. Averill JR. Personal control over aversive stimuli and its relationship to stress. *Psychological Bulletin* 1973; 80:288–303.
88. Moulton JM, Sweet DM, Temoshok L. Understanding attributions and health behavior changes in AIDS and ARC: Implications for interventions. In: Temoshock L, Baum A, eds. *Psychosocial Perspectives on AIDS. Etiology, Prevention, and Treatment.* Hillsdale, N.J.: Lawrence Erlbaum; 1990.
89. Brown I, Renwick R, Nagler M. The centrality of quality of life in health promotion and rehabilitation. In: Renwick R, Brown I, Nagler M, eds. *Quality of Life in Health Promotion and Rehabilitation. Conceptual Approaches, Issues, and Applications.* London: Sage Publications; 1996; 3–13.
90. Franchi D, Wenzel RP. Measuring health-related quality of life among patients infected with human immunodeficiency virus. *Clinical Infectious Diseases* 1998; 26:20–26.
91. Ware JE. Measuring patients' views: the optimum outcome measure. *British Medical Journal* 1993; 36:1429–1430.
92. Ross MW, Ryan L. The little deaths: perceptions of HIV, sexuality, and quality of life in gay men. In: Ross MW, ed. *HIV/AIDS and Sexuality.* New York: Harrington Press; 1995; 1–21.
93. Nilsson Schönnesson L. Quality of life among gay men and heterosexual women with HIV. A research study in progress.
94. Kaplan RM, Patterson TL, Kerner DN, *et al.* The quality of well-being scale in asymptomatic HIV-infected patients. *Quality of Life Research* 1997; 6(6):507–514.
95. Wu AW, Hays RD, Kelly S, *et al.* Applications of the Medical Outcome Study health-related quality of life measures in HIV/AIDS. *Quality of Life Research* 1997; 6:531–554.
96. Cella DF, McCain AJ, Peterman AH, *et al.* Development and validation of the Functional Assessment of Human Immundeficiency virus infection (FAHI) quality of life measurement. *Quality of Life Research* 1996; 5:450–463.
97. Holmes WC, Shea JA. A new HIV/AIDS-targeted quality of life (HAT-QoL) instrument. Development, reliability, and validity. *Medical Care* 1998; 36(2):138–154.
98. Fanning M, Emmot SD. Validation of a quality of life instrument for patients with HIV. (NHRDP Publication no. 6606-4334-AIDS). Ottawa, Ontario: *Health and Welfare Canada*; 1994.
99. Chuang H, Devins G, Hunsley J, *et al.* Psychosocial distress and well-being among gay and bisexual men with human immunodeficiency virus infection. *American Journal of Psychiatry* 1989; 146:876–880.
100. Cleary P, Fowler F, Weissman J, *et al.* Health-related quality of life in persons with acquired immune deficiency syndrome. *Medical Care* 1993; 31:300–314.
101. Holmes WC, Bix B, Meritz M, *et al.* Human immunodeficiency virus (HIV) infection and quality of life; the potential impact of Axis I psychiatric disorders in a sample of 95 HIV-seropositive men. *Psychosomatic Medicine* 1997; 59(2):187–192.

102. Rubin HC, Patterson TL, Atkinson JH, *et al.* Quality of life in people with depressive symptoms and HIV. International Conference on AIDS 1994; 10(1):194 (abstract no. PB0205)
103. Renwick R, Friedland J. Quality of life experienced by a sample of adults with HIV. In: Renwick R, Brown I, Nagler M, eds. *Quality of Life in Health Promotion and Rehabilitation. Conceptual Approaches, Issues, and Applications*. London: Sage Publications; 1996; 171–189.

II

Psychological Landscapes

7

The Existential Context

When we are confronted with a boundary situation[1] that threatens our physical and psychological survival such as HIV disease, we often become aware of the givens of existence and their importance to us. The ultimate concerns or givens of existence are meaning, death, freedom, and isolation.[2]

Within the health care system, however, there is a risk that the existential aspect of life is overlooked, as the dominant perspective on diseases (and health) is of a positivistic character. Tillich[3] argues that the concepts of health and disease are themselves existential, as disease represents the possibility and reality of life's distortion, and health may be seen as the conquering of disease. Thus, health/disease should not only be equated with longevity but should also include existential well-being.

As stated in Chapter 1, we regard the existential context to be one component of the psychological landscape within which the drama of HIV is dealt with. In this chapter we address each of the four ultimate existential concerns within a philosophical/existential frame of reference. We also highlight the givens from a general psychological/clinical lookout, including thoughts, feelings, and behavior that may take place when human beings encounter these concerns. The general description of the existential perspective is applied to HIV as it is reflected among those gay men with HIV who make up Dr. Schönnesson's psychotherapeutic material. As will be shown, each of the existential givens can be more or less salient and consciously experienced in various phases of the disease (the asymptomatic, mild, severe symptomatic, and the terminal phases). The significance of existential issues in the psychotherapeutic process is illuminated by the fact that all of the men in this study addressed these issues, in particular those related to dying and death. The intensity of the existential theme significantly increased over the disease phases.

MEANING

HIV-related threats and psychological issues may not only affect psychological functioning but also engender crisis in meaning of life. The individual's assumptive world or view of life is heavily attacked. It may become shattered as the person's sense of purpose or meaning with life, control, and self-worth is more or less violated. As a consequence, he may experience chaos. Depth, duration, and the character of the crisis may vary within the individual depending upon the kind of HIV-related threat or psychological issue he encounters.

Meaning of Life

From the existential perspective, the human being is thrown into a universe that has no meaning and his or her task is to construct his or her own meaning in life. Camus held that "the question of life's meaning is the most urgent question of all."[4] A common clinical phenomenon of today is people's encountering of senselessness, aimlessness, meaninglessness, and purposelessness. Within this context Frankl[5] talks about a crisis of meaninglessness as a symptom of low self-esteem, identity crisis, and depression. People may perceive an existential vacuum characterized by boredom, apathy, and emptiness. The experience of meaninglessness may also be a reflection of anxiety related to death, freedom, or isolation. One of many approaches to avoid the sense of meaninglessness is to engage in activities in a frantic way. Tom experiences that "if I don't have anything going or if I'm not in a love relationship, well then I'm not alive." Or in Tolstoy's words, "It is possible to live only as long as life intoxicates us"[2] (p. 481).

When we talk about meaning of life we often use the terms "meaning" and "purpose" interchangeably. However, within the existential context they have different connotations. Meaning refers to a cosmic meaning of some magical or spiritual ordering of the universe and whether life in general fits into some overall coherent pattern. Purpose is designated to intention, aim, or function. Despite this there is a reciprocity between the two concepts; a person who possesses a sense of meaning experiences life as having some purpose or function to be fulfilled.

Usually we do not ponder much about the meaning of life, but it is often related to everyday circumstances such as friends, family, work, and well-being. However, many gay men have long before HIV struggled with the existential concern of meaning in response to growing up as gay. The gay identity process as such challenges traditional norms, and gay men have to redefine meaning in the context of being gay to find meaning in their lives. White states:

> We could speak of that obligatory existentialism forced on people who must invent themselves.... Once one discovers one is gay one must choose everything from how to walk, dress and talk to where to live, with whom, and on what terms.... The nature of gay life is that it is philosophical.[6] (p. 16)

The meaning of life was a theme that about two-thirds of the men in this study brought up at some point in their therapeutic work. Yet, the data also revealed that when the person is very sick or dying there appears to be no room for existential questions such as the meaning in life, but existential guilt and quality of life take precedence. Meaning of life appeared to be mentioned and reflected upon in particular among those men who were in the asymptomatic phase. They dwelled upon it but usually the question left them with a question mark. Peter observes, "No, I don't really know what this is all about," or as Joseph notes, "I have no answer to my question." Frank concludes: "It has been important to me to discuss these matters but I am not sure I am that much wiser now than before." But there are exceptions. Like Harald who saw the purpose of his life as an endeavor for perfection. Another man, Jeffrey, talked about meaning in terms of being cosmic, spiritual, religious.

Why Do We Need Meaning?

Frankl[5] argued that the search for meaning is the basic need for human beings. He also proposed the assumption that the need for meaning or "the will to meaning" is a separate motivating power in personality as opposed to Freud's pleasure principle or the focus of self psychology on interrelationships.

Our search for meaning in life, which is an ongoing process, is based on our needs for overall perceptual frameworks and for a system of values or beliefs to interpret and make sense and order out of our lives and our place in the world. So we formulate our own assumptive worlds[7] or "a working model of the world."[8] Theoreticians suggest various explanatory models to understand the ways in which people create meaning or assumptive worlds. Baumeister[9] holds that people base their lives' meaning on four domains: (1) a sense of purpose; (2) a sense of morality or value; (3) a sense of being in control of our lives; and (4) a sense of self-worth. Janoff-Bulman[7] notes that the following core beliefs about life's meaning are shared by most people in the Western countries: First, the universe is just and fair; second, people can—and should—control the outcome of what happens to them; third, life events follow the rules of cause and effect and not randomness.

Peter expressed strong feelings of injustice about becoming infected: "I really don't deserve to be infected," and thus expressed a sense of being violated of his beliefs in a just world. He asked himself for quite some time, "What did I do to deserve this?" In his view of life HIV was a bad thing. Consequently, he must have been a "bad" person because he got HIV. Peter states:

> People get what they deserve. But honestly I don't understand what I have done wrong. I've always seen myself as a good and decent guy, but maybe I am not?

In other words, Peter's self-image was heavily shattered.

We think that both Baumeister's and Janoff-Bulman's perspectives bear similarities to the concept of view of life,[10] that is, general theories about man and the world, a system of beliefs and values indicating basic rules for life, and a basic attitude toward the world and other people.[11] Basic attitude refers to a mood that is either hopeful or trusting or one that is full of anguish and mistrust. This basic attitude plays an important role in the way HIV is integrated into one's life.

Hubert's childhood was extremely traumatic, leading to among others a sense of being unworthy, unloved, and unwanted as well as a great hesitance to trust anybody. Subsequently, Hubert feels very alone with his HIV infection; he would like to share his worries and concerns related to HIV with others, but he does not dare to out of fear of rejection. As Hubert states, "I was never of concern to anyone as a child, so why should that have changed just because I'm an adult?"

The Meaning of HIV Disease

The HIV-related crisis of meaning may raise existential questions such as Why did it happen? and Why me? The person tries to answer these questions in order to reconstrue or restore the basic, implicit assumptions (i.e., his view of life) he held about himself and the world prior to the traumatic event.[12] One aspect of this readjustment process is the search for meaning in the adverse experience,[13] that is, the individual's psychological need to find an explanation why the traumatic event, such as HIV infection, occurred in his life. One way to answer that question is through attributions.

Attribution theory[14] states that following a threatening or dramatic event, people will make attributions so as to understand, predict, and control their environment.[15] These psychological explanations of an illness can be attributed to the self, some other person, the environment, or chance. Historically, as Rosenberg[16] argues, there has been a desire to explain disease and death in terms of acts of will. In the late twentieth century the explanations have been replaced by a ruling morality on a healthy mind in a healthy body. Within such a perspective it becomes possible to think of disease as

> the effect of an individual's failure to act responsibly—to exercise, give up overeating, drinking and smoking, or to fight sexual addictions and sexual excess. If death can be indefinitely postponed by constant battle against a series of discrete attacks on the perfectible body, a battle led by the medical profession with the bodily disciplined rank and file of the healthy, then disease and death can be blamed on individuals who fail to live by the new norms. Death becomes a curable disease.[17] (p. 164)

HIV infection fits very well into the above description as it has been associated with personal responsibility, blame, and "the guilty" since it was first labeled as the "gay plague" in the early 1980s. Therefore, self-blame attributions and to what extent gay men have internalized this attitude are of particular interest. Various studies[18–22] confirm that many gay men have incorporated the self-blame label.

Interestingly enough, within the clinical context there were few men who asked themselves the question "Why me?" and who directly blamed themselves for being infected. But indirectly, it is possible to identify strokes of self-blame in quotes such as, "Why did I go to the sauna although I did know about HIV?" or "Why did I have sex with him, who I knew had HIV?" Such questions reflect a questioning of whether one's character or personality may have contributed to that person's becoming HIV seropositive. Most of the men attribute their HIV infection to chance. Quite a common remark is Benny's:

> I know there are people who accuse themselves for being HIV positive but I don't. Why should I? I know how I got infected and why I got it and when I got it is pure chance. And that's fine with me.

Minimal research has examined the relationship between self-blame (or other HIV-attribution theories for that matter) and psychological functioning. In Moulton et al. study[18] among gay men with AIDS and ARC (AIDS-related complex), holding oneself responsible for contracting HIV as well as self-blame were associated with distress among gay men with AIDS, but no such relationship was found among people with ARC. They also compared those who blamed themselves versus those who did not but no differences in distress were found in either the AIDS or ARC group. In another study, Clement and Nilsson Schönnesson[23] found that few of the gay men had exclusively incorporated the attribution of self-blame for their HIV infection. About one-third of them attributed "responsibility" to both self-blame and external factors. The investigators suggest that this co-existence may be understood in terms of ambivalence. On the one hand, the individual maintains that he does not "deserve" the infection and he projects all responsibility onto others but on the other hand he attributes the disease to his internal "preconditions" for contracting the infection. Self-blame attribution for contracting HIV was related to depressiveness and life dissatisfaction.

Another way that may help the person restore his sense of meaning in life is the kind of attribution (or representation) he assigns to HIV infection as such. These representations are ways to make sense of or to construe a psychological interpretation frame to or mentally depict HIV. Schwartzberg[24] identified ten representations (his own words) of HIV, similar to Lipowski's cognitive schema.[25] Schwartzberg also found that the men relied on a small number of these representations as the basis to rebuild their live's meaning. Below we make a short presentation of each of them.

Personal growth. HIV becomes an impetus to do something with one's life, to move forward, to make changes, to work with oneself.

Spiritual growth. To some it is "a nostalgic return to the church," for others spirituality becomes of greater priority, to others more of questioning, and to some HIV leads to a major reorientation of life in which religion comes to play a major role.

HIV as belonging. To some men this sense of belonging is related to close relationships, love relationships, and others find this belonging in a greater context, such as, the gay community, and thus strengthen their gay pride.

HIV as relief. HIV also has the capability to liberate. It may ease a burden of secrecy and become an impetus to come out as gay. At a deeper level,

Schwarzberg argues, HIV offers relief to some people "facing death can release you to face life"[24] (p. 51).

HIV as a strategy. HIV becomes a strategy to receive love, attention, acknowledgment, or recognition. It can also be a tool to get public attention. It is important to remember that this representation is not necessarily at a conscious level.

HIV as punishment. Some people see HIV as a punishment for an earlier sin or "crimes," such as that gay men are too sexual, too hedonistic, too indulgent.

HIV as contamination may be more salient right after the diagnosis.

HIV as confirmation of powerlessness. HIV confirms the way the individual sees himself in relation to the world—he is powerless against larger, uncontrollable forces, a kind of resignation. "It just happened," "If things happen, they happen." Life is expected to offer random, "capricious difficulties," and by some men HIV is viewed as an ordinary event, just one event among other hardships.

HIV as isolation. One may feel stronger bonds and belonging to other men with HIV but ostracized by the larger gay and straight communities.

HIV as irreparable loss. To many gay men HIV has meaning as an agent of massive sorrow. There are personal and communal losses and they blend together.

Some of these representations (e.g., punishment, irreparable loss, and powerlessness) come across as being negative to the individual's self-image. But at the same time these negative representations may serve an important purpose in that they uphold a framework of meaning in life. The negative impact on self-image may be regarded by some men as "better" than seeing the world as meaningless or as random.

To what extent are these HIV attributions found in the psychotherapeutic context? Most of them are recognizable but the least frequent one was spiritual growth. Yet, two of the men talked about HIV in those terms, albeit quite differently. Leon, who had a strong faith since childhood, during a phase of his psychotherapeutic work, was quite occupied with questioning his religiosity. He experienced that HIV had led him to reflect upon whether his religiosity was "genuine," or as he put it himself, "of a neurotic character." To Carl HIV became an impetus to direct himself toward faith, and eventually he converted to another Christian denomination. It should be noted that Sweden is significantly more secular than the United States, and that formal Christianity is much less common. However, this difference is one of emphasis. The clinical material showed that reflections related to spirituality rather than religiosity were quite common.

The psychotherapeutic notes of the gay men also presented additional representations than those described by Schwarzberg. The most frequent HIV representations were limitation, finitude, punishment, persecution, and imprisonment. Most of the gay men, regardless of disease phase, viewed HIV as a limitation in terms of time, social, and behavioral activities. In the asymptomatic phase limitation was reinforced by the view of HIV as finitude ("annihilation," "death sentence," "a bomb") and irreparable loss. One could argue that limitation, finitude, and irreparable loss all symbolize a cul-de-sac, which could be interpreted as the symbol of the final boundary of life, death.

The attribution of "prison" on the other hand was only mentioned in the severe symptomatic phase. The perception of "prison" is realistic in the severe symptomatic phase in that the symptoms do limit the person's activities and he may perceive himself as being in a prison. But the "prison" attribution could also be interpreted as a punishment for having "committed a crime," that is, self-blame.

In the mild symptomatic and the dying phases HIV infection represented a persecutor. In the dying phase the person is haunted in a realistic way by a bad object, HIV, that is to kill him. In the mild symptomatic phase the persecutor representation was reinforced by the one of punishment. It could be speculated that when the first HIV-related symptoms appear, HIV becomes concrete and a reality to the individual, leading to a sense of being persecuted by the "wicked." The persecution might also be perceived as a punishment.

To summarize, it seems like the HIV representations changed over the disease phases from a concrete perception of death to psychological representations of prison and persecutor.

DEATH

Dying and Death

> *Of all the world's wonders, which is the most wonderful? That no man, though he sees others dying all around him, believes that he himself will die.*
>
> —Yudhishtara answers Dharma from "The Mahabharata"

Dying and death are two phenomena that both frighten and fascinate human beings. Death is the most obvious given of existence as it is inevitable. We exist now, but death will come and there is no escape from it. Although we all know—intellectually—that we will die one day, it is still hard to accept that fact.

On both an individual and a cultural level, we consume a lot of energy to avoid and deny thoughts and feelings about death. Death is taboo. We are even hesitant to use the words "He has died" but rather voice words like "He passed away" or, "He is gone."

Death signifies different meanings to different people.[26] To some death is absurd, meaningless, and equal to annihilation, torment, or solitude. To others, death is encountered with positive aspects, such as belief in an afterlife or immortality, reunion with loved ones who are already dead, reabsorption into cosmic unity, an escape from a miserable life, a liberator. But most people are ambivalent about death. A somewhat neutral attitude is reflected in the following statement from Hubert: "After death there is nothing. When I am dead I am dead. Period."

From a philosophical/existential perspective, life and death are psychologically merged into each other in that death enriches rather than impoverishes life. The Stoics as well as contemporary writers stress that learning to live well is learning to die well. Conversely the art of dying is the art of living, "the dignity we seek in dying must be found in the dignity with which we have lived our lives"[27] (p. 268). St. Augustine (as cited in Yalom[2]) expressed the idea that "It is only in the face of death that man's self is born" and to quote Yalom[28] "to live fully one must accept that it ends." Heidegger[29] has explored how "the idea of death may save man." He arrived at the insight that there are two fundamental modes of existing in the world: (1) a state of forgetfulness of being or (2) a state of mindfulness of being. Ordinarily we live in the first state, in which we surrender ourselves to a concern about the *way* that things are. Heidegger means, that the state of forgetfulness of being is a mode in which one is unaware of one's authorship of one's life and world. In the other state, the state of mindfulness of being, one marvels *that* things are. In these modes one remains mindful of the fragility of being and of one's responsibility for one's own being. In order to be able to live life in such an authentic fashion, we have to integrate the *idea* of death. As Heidegger emphasizes, the idea of death does not sentence us to pessimism, just on the contrary. It enhances our pleasure in the living of life and acts as a spur to live more authentic life modes.[29]

Another philosophical aspect of death is its close link to time. "The thought of death presupposes time"[30] (p. 22). Time is something we usually take for granted and we do not really have a sense of time going by. In our Western culture time has become "a commodity, measured in minutes and hours rather than in depth of experience"[31] (p. 223). Yet, the comprehension of time, that is, the ability to connect the present with the past and the future, is an important element of our existence. To people with HIV—at least upon until now—the future (i.e., chronological time) has been ripped off and so has its certainty and stability of ongoingness.[32]

Feigenberg[30] says that time can be differentiated between chronological and existential time. Whereas chronological time refers to the idea that time is a linear and everlasting process, existential time is the expression of the personal meaning of what happens to a human being in the present. In the process of dying the passage of time creates anxiety and the perception of chronological time alters and disintegrates in favor of existential time. A dying person is in the situation of being in the process of dying and time simply *is*.

One aspect of death, and a controversial one, is physician-assisted suicide and euthanasia. The former designates to the person's request, in advance, for a prescription for barbiturates to have "the means" available when he considers his life intolerable. The person is usually medically stable when he asks his physician for the help. Euthanasia means that the physician terminates life at the explicit request of the patient by administrating a lethal drug when he is actively dying. Both forms of end-of-life measures are still taboo and legally and ethically complicated. In the United States and in Sweden it is illegal to actively assist a suicide as well as to perform euthanasia. The sensitivity of the topic is also reflected in the paucity of works on euthanasia and assisted death within the HIV research forum. Starace and Ogden[33] point out in their report from the Vancouver AIDS conference in 1996 that only three presentations (of which one was a case report) specifically addressed the end-of-life issues of euthanasia. Dutch studies[34,35] indicate that the incidence of euthanasia/assisted suicide among AIDS patients in the Netherlands is between 22% and 26%. That figure is far greater than that for Dutch patients with cancer, among whom 7% choose euthanasia. Another study[36] documented that 2.7% of all AIDS deaths in British Columbia were the result of euthanasia/assisted suicide (although such figures are probably underestimated). The same study also showed that the majority (83%) of the persons with HIV/AIDS considered euthanasia/assisted suicide as a possible choice. Almost half of the respondents (44%) had had prepared plans for an assisted suicide.

In Dr. Schönnesson's case load a few men have told her about their views on assisted suicide, as illustrated by the following quote from Adam:

> When the day comes when I can't take care of myself anymore and my body is just a wreck and I'm lost as a person, then I have my provisions at home.

Some men have asked to have their living wills included in their record file. David says:

> Make a note in my file that when the day comes when I am really sick I don't want the doctors to put me onto life-extending treatment. And I don't want to have an autopsy.

In the psychotherapeutic setting the theme of death is not only related to or brought up in the terminal phase (phase 4) of life. As stated earlier, all the gay men in Dr. Schönnesson's note material talked about death, in particular during the first three phases of the disease. Given the reality of many gay men—at least in urban areas—with the likelihood of knowing others who have HIV, are sick, or dying being high, it is not surprising that death thoughts occurred for example at the death of a friend or lover. Dr. Schönnesson's experience is that when a friend or lover dies it stirs up emotions and reflections related to one's own death. To quote Michael, whose lover died: "Who is going to take care of me when I get sick and be at my bedside when I am dying?"

Another context within which thoughts of death occurred was when the men were preparing (in their fantasy or in reality) their own funeral arrangements and/or their will. This happened in particular in the asymptomatic (phase 1) and the mild symptomatic (phase 2) phases. This could be a reflection of a way to "familiarize" oneself with death and to make it real, as it is still abstract and perceived as a threat in those disease phases. Maybe it is a way to start integrating death into life?

In the second, mild symptomatic, phase of the disease some of the men expressed a longing for death. After-death thoughts were a theme to some of those men who entered the severe symptomatic phase. It could be speculated that when impending death becomes real and obvious, the individual also becomes aware of his death anxiety. The after-death thoughts could thus be interpreted as a manifestation of the illusion of immortality.

As mentioned earlier in this chapter, death can also indirectly be spoken about by means of HIV representations. The vast majority of the gay men who still had an intact immune system and no symptoms talked about HIV in terms of annihilation, death sentence, and a time bomb. These representations can all be interpreted as a manifestation of finitude. Later in the disease those words were replaced by limitation, which is also indirectly a synonym of death—our life is limited by death.

Death Fear and Anxiety

Fear and anxiety surround death. The primitive dread of death is part of the fabric of being and is formed early in life and it resides in the unconscious. [2] There are disagreements whether death fear is a natural thing for man. One argument holds that fear of death is not a natural thing for man but something that society creates.[37] It argues that if the child "has good maternal experiences [he or she] will develop a sense of basic security and will not be subject to morbid fears of losing support, of being annihilated, or the like" (Tiertz as cited by Becker,[37] pp. 13–14). The other argument goes that fear of death is natural and is present in everyone. It is the basic fear that influences all others, a fear from which no one is immune. Zilboorg (as cited by Becker[37]) says that most people think that death fear is absent because it rarely shows its face. But beneath all appearances fear of death is universally present.

The concept of death fear is often used synonymously with death anxiety. What exactly is it that we fear of death? Usually when we talk about death fear we refer to fears related to death,[38] such as the dying process or what comes after death.[39] This mode is reflected in Templer and Geer's[40] look at the relationship between death anxiety and HIV disease. They suggest that death anxiety may emerge from either fear of pain and suffering associated with dying or from fear about what happens after life. From an existential point of view, however, "ceasing to be" is centrally the fear of death.[38,40] Kierkegaard[41] made a clear distinction between anxiety and fear. Anxiety refers to a fear of losing oneself and becoming nothingness. Fear on the other hand, is fear of *some* thing. Anxiety, according to Yalom, cannot be located and

> a fear that can neither be understood nor located cannot be confronted and becomes more terrible still: it begets a feeling of helplessness, which invariably generates further anxiety.[2] (p. 43)

Similar ideas can be found in self psychologist Kohut's[42] concept of disintegration anxiety, which is, according to Kohut, the basic and deepest anxiety man can experience. What is feared is ceasing to be a human self, that is, a psychological death or a loss of humanness. Kohut maintains that disintegration anxiety is closer to death anxiety than to what Freud designated the fear of loss of love. Whereas Freud viewed death anxiety as stemming from castration or separation anxieties, Klein and existential psychodynamic-oriented psychotherapists consider the death anxiety as the original source of anxiety. Self-psychology deems that various forms of anxieties are expressions of disintegration anxiety.

It is rare to encounter the existential death anxiety in clinical work as it is usually covered up and masked with various denial-based defense mechanisms. The disguised transformation of death anxiety may take the form of the thought that one will be forgotten. But sometimes the raw death anxiety bursts into the consciousness. Stephen told the therapist the following nightmare, which he interpreted as "now I know what death anxiety is all about." The dream takes place in the Inca era. Stephen is carried in a chair up to a fire to be sacrificed. Along the side there are men holding tall candle lights. He reaches the hill with the fire, he shivers from fear, and the men put him into the fire.

To conduct empirical research related to death anxiety has proven to be an arduous task. Most studies have measured conscious attitudes toward death or conscious manifest death anxiety. Non-HIV related studies have identified among other things that highly religious people have less death anxiety and people in ill health have lower death anxiety than do healthy people.[40] People with mental illness, depression, high levels of anxiety, or maladjustment tend to have higher death anxiety.[40] Research on death anxiety among gay men with HIV is very sparse, but existing findings diverge from the general ones. One study[43] found that gay men with AIDS had higher death anxiety scores than noninfected gay men. Findings from another study indicated a positive correlation between death anxiety and HIV progression "perhaps because HIV-infected gay men get less support from family and religious congregation as death approaches"[44] (p. 3). Among the male participants with HIV, death anxiety was positively associated with religion. The researchers interpreted the finding as a reflection that most Christian denominations have regarded homosexuality as a sin to be punished by God after death. The same study also showed a very strong link between death anxiety and general anxiety and depression.

Templer[45] argues that the individual's past experience with death and the general state of a person's psychological well-being determine the level of death anxiety. Others have developed a more complex model for understanding contributing factors to death fear. Tomer and Eliason,[26] for example, suggest that there are three determinants of death anxiety; past-related regret (the individual feels guilty for not having accomplished what he expected to accomplish), future-related regret (realization that the future necessary for completion of goals and tasks may no longer be available), and meaningfulness of death. According to their model a person will experience high death anxiety when he feels much past and future regret or perceives death as meaningless.

Death-Defense Strategies

The fear of death is of such a magnitude that it has to be repressed in one or another way. "If this fear was constantly conscious, we should be unable to function normally" (Zilboorg as cited by Becker,[37] p. 17). In our attempts to cope with these fears we may construct adaptive defenses such as denial, repression, displacement, and rationalization. Another strategy to circumvent the reality of death and its related anxiety is to immerse oneself into symbolic immortality. Lifton[46] has described five modes. First, the biological mode—living on through one's progeny; second, the theological mode—living on in a different, higher plane of existence; third, the creative mode—living on through one's work; fourth, the mode of eternal nature—one survives through rejoining the swirling life forces of nature; and fifth, the experiential transcendent mode—through "losing oneself" in a state so intense that time and death disappear and one lives in the "continuous present." The symbolic immortality modes that have been met in Dr. Schönnesson's clinical practice are creative ones in terms of being active in the Body Positive group or writing or painting. An example of the eternal nature is illustrated in Paul's words: "one is transformed into energy and then one returns to earth. It's like a circle." The biological mode is discussed by some from the perspective of lost fatherhood and its concomitant sense of loss and mourning. These men mean that because no child will survive them, they will not "continue to live." In other words, children can be viewed as a way of being immortal.

We also develop defense strategies, such as the belief in the existence of an ultimate rescuer and a delusional belief in one's specialness and inviolability.[2] The former is assumed to be less effective than the specialness defense. Generally we perform traces of them both (in combination with other defenses as well). Both beliefs can be adaptive defense strategies, but they may also be overloaded and break down. The irrational belief in a rescuer is probably most challenged by a serious/fatal disease. It is Dr. Schönnesson's experience that the belief in the rescuer or protector becomes more salient when the gay men display a series of HIV-related symptoms and perhaps are also hospitalized. The physician is more or less consciously assigned the magical role of a rescuer. It becomes important to the client to "behave well" in fear of being abandoned by him or her, because if abandoned the protection of death is gone. In psychodynamic language we could say that the rescuer role is similar to idealization, which is further elaborated on in Chapter 9. In one's capacity as a therapist it is quite common to be idealized. David, who had been on the waiting list to receive therapy for some time, said when he came to his first therapeutic session, "I have been fighting for quite some time to get to you, and now when I'm here it's almost like coming to God."

With respect to specialness, Yalom makes a distinction between its rational and death defensive dimensions. The rational side is that any individual is special in that he has special qualities and gifts, that he has a unique life history, and that no one who had ever lived is just like him. But we (some more than others) also have an irrational sense of specialness.

> It [specialness] is one of our chief methods of denying death, and the part of our mind whose task it is to mollify death terror generates the irrational belief that we are invulnerable—that unpleasant things like aging and death may be the lot of others but not our lot, that we exist beyond law, beyond human and biological destiny.[47] (p. 149)

It goes without saying that when an individual is confronted with HIV, this illusion of specialness is badly shattered.

In the terminal phase the person also tries additional ways to protect himself from being overwhelmed by death fear. Examples of such strategies are the affectionate care from family or friends, the conviction of meeting dead friends and families, to marvel at one's rich life, memory of fusion, to be united with nature. Death is far more difficult to face when the individual does not have such consolations or when they feel deprived of human contacts they do need.[48]

Death and Personal Change

In Tolstoy's[49] *War and Peace*, Pierre is captured by Napoleon and sentenced to death. He watches the execution of five men in line, him being the sixth. He prepares to die and at the last moment he is unexpectedly reprieved. This experience transforms Pierre. Death salience may thus cause an increased sense of life vulnerability and lead to personal positive change in, for example, self concept and self-esteem but also in view of life. Like Yalom's[2] description of patients with terminal cancer many of the gay men describe a reassessment of life priorities, increased sensibility to one's needs and wishes, and a stronger self.

FREEDOM

Meaning and death are not the only ultimate concerns that are "a part of, and an inescapable part, of the human being's existence in the world"[2] (p. 8). Freedom is another given of existence that we are confronted with and it encompasses to the philosopher a wide terrain. In this section we focus on only one aspect of freedom, namely, responsibility. In its existential sense responsibility means that each individual is the creator of his world, life design, choices, and actions. But it also implies an awareness of one's responsibility. One of the gay men, Robert, talked about his existential responsibility in terms of having HIV: "I made the choice to have unprotected sex with him. I could have said no, but I did not. And I did it against my ideals."

In this quote we can also detect existential guilt in terms of him betraying his own ideals and moral code. Guilt is the dark presence of responsibility. Within the existential frame of reference guilt assumes a somewhat different meaning from traditional psychoanalytic theories.[2] Traditional guilt refers to real or fantasized transgressions against another or against some moral or social code. Kierkegaard[50] and later Tillich[51] called attention to another source of guilt—existential guilt. It is defined in terms of transgression against oneself. Tillich says:

> Man's being is not only given to him but also demanded of him. He is responsible for it; literally, he is required to answer, if he is asked, what he has made of himself. He who asks him is his judge, namely he himself. The situation produces the anxiety, which in relative terms is the anxiety of guilt, in absolute terms the anxiety of self-rejection or condemnation. Man is asked to make of himself what he is supposed to become, to fulfil his destiny. In every act of moral, self-affirmation man contributes to the fulfillment of his destiny, to the actualization of what he potentially is.[51] (p. 52)

To some men it is very painful to realize that they have not achieved what they wanted to do with their lives. "So this is all my life is about?" or "Life really cheated me." Others may not have put up any life goals, which they now, closer to death, become aware of, often leading to quilt feelings. Larry mourned: "Well, I can't be proud of myself. I wouldn't say that I have made the most of it."

If we accept the existential perspective of having responsibility for our lives it also implies that we have to make decisions and to act upon them. However, human beings find it difficult to decide when we cannot predict our decision's potential consequences. We always run the risk of making the wrong decision. Why is it then difficult to make a decision—to commit oneself to something? There may be many (conscious as well as unconscious) reasons but probably the strongest one is that to decide one thing always means to relinquish something else.

> Decisions are painful because they signify the limitations of possibilities; and the more one's possibilities are limited, the closer one is brought to death.... The reality of limitation is a threat to one of our chief modes of coping with existential anxiety; the delusion of specialness—that, though others may be subject to limitations, one is exempt, special, and beyond natural law.[2] (p. 318)

We would argue that existential responsibility is important to acknowledge within the HIV realm to better understand why individuals may have difficulties in making decisions regarding, for example, self-disclosure and medical treatment. Disclosure is one example of a situation where the person has to make a decision. The individual may hesitate because he cannot anticipate or know for sure about the consequences of the disclosure. On the other hand, if the individual decides not to disclose his HIV status that also implies consequences. As stated above, decisions limit other possibilities and limits are in its deepest sense equal to death. In other words, ambivalence related to self-disclosure cannot only be understood in rational terms but attention also has to be paid to existential concerns.

EXISTENTIAL ISOLATION

Many people talk about their fear of interpersonal isolation—to be rejected or abandoned by others. We suggest that underlying this fear is an even deeper fear, namely, the fear of existential isolation. The basic isolation is:

> An isolation that persists despite the most gratifying engagement with other individuals and despite consummate self-knowledge and integration.... [It] refers to an unbridgeable gulf between oneself and any other being ... a separation between the individual and the world.[2] (p. 355)

When the individual experiences existential isolation he may describe it as "there is no one else there but me" or "it is like the world is fading away." But isolation also indicates our fundamental isolation, that is, each of us enters existence alone and must depart from it alone. Aloneness means here, that the individual has to experience birth and death all on his own. As to death, there is no "stand in" for my death, no one can die my death for me. I have to experience it all by myself. This fundamental isolation is fearful, which is clearly illustrated by the following fantasy as described by Kenneth:

> I'm lying in the coffin, but there is a hole through which I can stick out my hand. You're standing next to the coffin, dressed in white, and I put out my hand to reach your hand and you take it. It's such a consolation.

Fromm[52] believed that existential isolation, the basic separateness and its concomitant sense of helplessness, is our primary source of anxiety. But we try to find ways to protect ourselves from coming in touch with these feelings. The strong focus on intimate relationships as "a touchstone of health and happiness"[53] often functions, according to Yalom,[2] as a means to keep existential isolation within manageable bounds. But love, says Yalom, "does not take away our separateness—that is a given of existence and can be faced but never erased"[2] (p. 370). He and Fromm appear to agree that love is "our best mode of coping with the pain of separateness"[2] (p. 370).

EXISTENTIAL ANXIETY

As a response to the insight into the inescapable limitations of existence, aloneness, and vulnerability, the individual may experience existential anxiety.

This kind of anxiety reaction has to be separated from neurotic anxiety, which is generated from unconscious, internal, repressed conflicts. However, the nucleus of all anxiety is the fear of being alone, separated, and helpless. These feelings, according to psychoanalytic theory, originate from the child's experience of loss, aloneness, and helplessness. These experiences will eventually constitute a psychological base for adult life crisis. Another way to put it is that the child's separation anxiety corresponds to the adult's experience of a total helplessness toward universal mortality. Although existential and neurotic anxiety stem from different sources, there is a link between the two.

> The existential anxiety of death, personal responsibility, guilt, and questions about the meaning of life can be reinforced, colored, and intermittently exceeded by a non-worked through internal conflict from the first years of life. Worries of annihilation, that are embedded in the consciousness of one's own death, can be affected disproportionately strong by early losses and non-healed grief.[54] (p. 82)

SUMMARY

HIV raises existential issues within a philosophical frame of reference, usually relating to death, freedom, isolation, and meaning in life. While these are not necessarily clinical, they are an integral part of the psychotherapeutic process and represent one of the components of the individual psychological landscape within which the threats and psychological issues of HIV disease are dealt with.

REFERENCES

1. Jaspers K. Cited in Yalom I. *Existential Psychotherapy*. New York: Basic Books; 1980.
2. Yalom I. *Existential Psychotherapy*. New York: Basic Books; 1980.
3. Tillich P. *The Meaning of Health. Essays in Existentialism, Psychoanalysis, and Religion*. Chicago: Exploration Press; 1984.
4. Camus A. Cited in Jaffe A. *The Myth of Meaning in the Work of C. Jung*. London: Hodden & Stoughton, 1970.
5. Frankl V. *Man's Search for Meaning: An Introduction to Logotherapy*. New York: Simon and Schuster; 1962.
6. White E. *State of Desire: Travels in Gay America*. New York: EP Dutton; 1980.
7. Janoff-Bulman R. *Shattered Assumptions. Towards a New Psychology of Trauma*. New York: Free Press; 1995.
8. Bowlby J. *Attachment and Loss*. Vol. I: *Attachment*. London: Hogarth; 1969.
9. Baumeister RF. *Meaning of Life*. New York: Guilford; 1991.
10. Kallenberg K. *View-of-Life in a Crisis: An Empirical Study*. Örebro: Doxa; 1987.
11. Stifoss-Hanssen H, Kallenberg K. *Existential Questions and Health*. Report 1996:3, Swedish Council for Planning and Coordination of Research.
12. Janoff-Bulman R, Frieze JH. A theoretical perspective for understanding reactions to victimization. *Journal of Social Issues* 1983; 39:1–17.

13. Taylor SE. Adjustment to threatening events—A theory of cognitive adaptation. *American Psychologist* 1983; 41:1161–1173.
14. Kelley HH. Attribution theory in social psychology. In: Levine D, ed. *Nebraska Symposium on Motivation*. Lincoln: University of Nebraska Press; 1976; 192–238.
15. Wong PTP, Weiner B. When people ask "why" questions, and the heuristics of attributional search. *Journal of Personality and Social Psychology* 1981; 40:650–663.
16. Rosenberg C. Cited in Weeks J. *Invented Moralities. Sexual Values in an Age of Uncertainty*. New York: Columbia University Press; 1995.
17. Weeks J. *Invented Moralities. Sexual Values in an Age of Uncertainty*. New York: Columbia University Press; 1995.
18. Moulton JM, Sweet DM, Temoshok L. Understanding attributions and health behavior changes in AIDS and ARC: Implications for interventions. In: Temoshok L, Baum A. *Psychosocial Perspectives on AIDS Ethiology, Prevention, and Treatment*. Hillsdale, New Jersey: Lawrence Erlbaum; 1990; 191–200.
19. Barrett RL. Counseling gay men with AIDS: Human dimensions. *Journal of Counseling and Development* 1989; 67:573–575.
20. Ross MW, Rosser BS. Psychological issues in AIDS-related syndromes. *Patient Education and Counseling* 1988; 11:17–28.
21. Dilley JW, Ochitill HN, Perl M, *et al.* Findings in psychiatric consultations with patients with acquired immune deficiency syndrome. *American Journal of Psychiatry* 1995; 142:82–86.
22. Hirsch DA, Enlow RW. The effects of the acquired immune deficiency syndrome on gay lifestyle and the gay individual. *Annals of the New York Academy of Science* 1984; 437:273–282.
23. Clement U, Nilsson Schönnesson L. Subjective HIV attribution theories, coping, and psychological functioning among homosexual men with HIV. *AIDS Care* 1998; 10(3):355–364.
24. Schwartzberg S. *A Crisis of Meaning. How Gay Men Are Making Sense of AIDS*. New York: Oxford University Press; 1996.
25. Lipowski ZJ. Physical illness, the individual and the coping process. *Psychiatric Medicine* 1970; 1:91–102.
26. Tomer A, Eliason G. Toward a comprehensive model of death anxiety. *Death Studies* 1996; 20:343–365.
27. Nuland SB. *How We Die. Reflections on Life's Final Chapter*. New York: Vintage Books; 1992.
28. Branfman F. A matter of life and death. The *Salon* interview with Irvin Yalom; 1996.
29. Heidegger M. *Being and Time*. New York: Harper & Row; 1962.
30. Feigenberg L. *Terminal Care. Friendship Contracts with Dying Cancer Patients*. New York: Brunner & Mazel; 1980.
31. Van Deurzen-Smith E. *Existential Counselling in Practice*. London: Sage Publications; 1997.
32. Klitzman R. *Being Positive: The Lives of Men and Women with HIV*. Chicago: Ivan R. Dee; 1997.
33. Starace F, Ogden RD. Suicidal behaviors and euthanasia. *AIDS Care* 1997; 9(1):106–108.
34. Laane HM. The epidemiology of euthanasia and assisted suicide among PWAs in Amsterdam. Oral presentation, abstract WeD 240, 11th International Conference of AIDS, Vancouver, Canada; 1996.
35. Bindels PJ, Krol A, van Ameijden EJ, *et al.* Euthanasia and physician-assisted suicide among homosexual men with AIDS in the Netherlands. 3rd conference on retro and opportunistic infections, Jan. 28–Feb. 1, 1996; 152.
36. Ogden RD. Euthanasia and AIDS in British Columbia. Oral presentation, abstract WeD 241, 11th International Conference of AIDS, Vancouver, Canada; 1996.
37. Becker E. The terror of death. In: Williamson JB, Sheidman ES, eds. *Death: Current Perspectives* (4th ed.). Mountain View, California: Mayfield Publishing; 1995.
38. Kastenbaum R, Aisenberg R. *Psychology of Death*. New York: Springer; 1972.
39. Choron J. *Modern Man and Mortality*. New York: Macmillan; 1964.

40. Templer DI, Geer RD. Death anxiety and HIV disease. *Focus. A Guide to AIDS Research and Counseling*. 1996; 11(12):1–4.
41. Kierkegaard S. *The Concept of Dread*. Princeton, N.J.: Princeton University Press; 1944.
42. Kohut H. *How Does Analysis Cure?* Chicago: University of Chicago Press; 1984.
43. Franks K, Templer DI, Cappelletty G, *et al.* Exploration of death anxiety as a function of religious variables in gay men with and without AIDS. *Omega* 1990–1991; 22(1):43–49.
44. Hintze J, Templer DI, Cappelletty G, *et al.* Death depression and death anxiety in HIV-infected males. *Death Studies* 1993; 17(4):333–341.
45. Templer DI. Two factor theory of death anxiety: A note. *Essence* 1976; 1(1):91–93.
46. Lifton RJ. The sense of immortality: On death and the continuity of life. In: Lifton R and Olson E, eds. *Explorations in Psychohistory*. New York: Simon & Schuster; 1974; 271–288.
47. Yalom ID. *Love's Executioner and Other Tales of Psychotherapy*. New York: Harper Perennial, A Division of HarperCollins Publishers; 1989.
48. Dreifuss-Kattan E. *Cancer Stories. Creativity and Self-Repair*. Hillsdale, N.J.: Analytic Press; 1990.
49. Tolstoy L. *War and Peace*. New York: Modern Library; 1931.
50. Kierkegaard S. *The Sickness unto Death*. New York: Doubleday Anchor Books; 1941.
51. Tillich P. *The Courage to Be*. New Haven, CT: Yale University Press; 1952.
52. Fromm E. *The Art of Loving*. New York: Bantam Books; 1956.
53. Storr A. *Solitude. A Return to the Self*. New York: Ballantine Books; 1988.
54. Wikström O. *Den outgrundliga människan*. Stockholm: Natur och Kultur; 1991.

8

HIV Adaptation Processes

In Chapter 7 we discussed the existential context as being one of the components of the psychological landscape of HIV. The second component of the individual psychological landscape is HIV adaptation processes. In this chapter, we first address the concept of adaptation processes followed by three clinical vignettes to illustrate different adaptation processes of the HIV scenario.

Symbolically the life situation of a person with HIV can be pictured in the following way: his well-known, familiar ground is changed into a more or less new and unknown one. The person with HIV is confronted with the question: How am I to become familiar with this new ground, to feel confident in it, and to make it a part of myself? The overall question is: How can I achieve at least temporarily psychological and sexual well-being and carry on a satisfying and meaningful life that carries a sense of quality of life? The answers to these questions are unfolded in the individual's subjective HIV adaptation process. In other words, we suggest that quality of life is the ultimate goal of the adaptation process. However, it appears to be more accurate to talk about adaptation processes, as the person with HIV is faced with various HIV-related threats and psychological issues in the course of the disease. Thus, he needs to adapt to different crises, events, or situations that may be more or less taxing on him. Depending upon the adaptation process of a given crisis, event, or situation it exerts an influence on psychological functioning and quality of life, which may be affected in a positive or a negative way. Moreover, we suggest that the way the adaptation unfolds in certain threats and issues is more important than others to achieve a sense of an overall quality of life. This varies between individuals. In other words, neither psychological functioning nor quality of life is a fixed phenomenon but both are highly personal matters.

THE CONCEPT OF ADAPTATION PROCESS

We can identify two common approaches to describe the individual's adaptation process. The psychosocial variables model studies which ways the HIV infection exerts influence on the individual's psychological functioning over the disease phases and which psychosocial factors facilitate or impede the maintenance of psychological well-being over time. The most common theoretical model being used is, however, the five-stage model of grief.[1] It is aimed at describing the emotional reactions (denial, isolation, anger, bargaining, depression) and the coming to terms with (acceptance of) dying and death. Other stage crisis models focus mainly on the acute phase of emotional reactions to a crisis, for example, a disease diagnosis. According to these models, the emotional reactions disrupt the individual's psychic equilibrium. In order to restore it, the person has to pass through stages, such as the shock stage, the reaction stage, the working-through stage, and finally reaching the new orientation stage. However, no empirical studies support stage models among gay men with HIV.[2] Both the psychosocial variables model and stage crisis model run the risk of being perceived in a normative or hierarchical way. They tend to give the impression that there is a "right" or "normal" way to react or respond to a threat or psychological issues, that one approach is "better" or more "mature" than others. For those people with HIV who believe that they are not reacting in the "right" way, feelings of guilt or being abnormal may be evoked.

However, we would argue that neither of the two approaches described above does justice to the complexity of psychological and social mechanisms involved in the adaptation processes. We therefore suggest a theoretical framework, in which the HIV adaptation processes are viewed as a spiral model considering the reoccurring character of HIV-related threats and psychological issues. Further we argue that HIV adaptation processes can be understood as a function of psychological metabolism; in other words metabolizing is necessary to achieve adaptation.[3]

The concept of metabolizing is used here as a metaphor to describe an individual's active (more or less consciously) internal process of coming to grips with a given HIV threat or psychological issue. Every time the person is confronted with one, it may evoke psychological and cognitive chaos accompanied by a range of, and often a combination of, emotions. The extent to which the individual's psychological equilibrium and sense of self are threatened and manifested in psychological distress are dependent on the person's life history, personality, and current life context. Based on life history and personality, the individual develops his repertoire of HIV-related psychological, social, and cognitive tools, such as coping, social support, subjective meaning to HIV, attribution to the HIV infection, and perceived control of the HIV progression. By means of these tools and his personality the actual threat or psychological issue and its concomitant emotions are metabolized cognitively and mentally in terms of being incorporated, contained, and digested. The aim of psychological metabolism is to bring an ordering out of the chaos and in that way to restore the disrupted equilibrium and consequently minimize feelings of psychological suffering. However, the person's metabolizing is not always constructive to him in terms of reducing the chaotic scenario. Regardless of the "success" of the psychological metabolism, it has to be kept in mind that a given metabolizing makes sense and can be understood within the context of the individual's life conditions.

Yet, the individual HIV adaptation process is complicated by the fact that the self, which plays an important role in the adaptation process, may be more or less destabilized by, among others, the HIV-related threats and issues. Therefore, the individual may have to struggle more or less simultaneously not only with adapting to HIV threats and issues but also with restoring his shattered self. We therefore suggest that the HIV-disease adaptation processes interact with the self-adaptation processes, which will be addressed in Chapter 9.

The proposed theoretical framework is illustrated by means of two types of metabolizing patterns with respect to the HIV diagnosis. They were identified in a study among gay men with HIV conducted by Nilsson Schönnesson[4] and are based on two empirically identified coping styles (avoidant and self-assertive) and their statistical significant associations with personality and psychosocial tools. The avoidant metabolizing pattern was characterized by, on the one hand, emotional and cognitive avoidance of the HIV reality and hopes that it would disappear in a magical way, and, on the other hand, by depressive ruminations of becoming sick and a low perceived progression control. The infection was seen as a punishment or a weakness. There was also a self-reproach to the HIV infection, and the avoidant metabolizing encompassed a poor social support network. The pattern was found in a personality profile characterized by relationship difficulties and social withdrawal, a negative self-image, and elements of guilt feelings. The avoidant metabolizing pattern was associated with psychological distress in terms of depressiveness, sexual, and psychosomatic symptoms.

The self-assertive metabolizing displayed quite another pattern. It was distinguished by a positive self-esteem, trust in one's inner resources, and a fighting spirit attitude to influence the progression. HIV was regarded as a challenge and attributed to destiny. There was also a sense of control of HIV progression in terms of having access to a variety of coping strategies. The personality profile displayed a positive self-image and the capacity to initiate and maintain close, intimate relationships, as reflected in their broad social network and support system.

CLINICAL VIGNETTES

The three following case vignettes illustrate different adaptation processes of the HIV scenario. It is not possible to talk about "typical" cases and therefore these are not a "representative sample" of the 38 gay men from this study. However, each of them illuminates stories of living and dying with HIV and the renarratization of the disease.

Barry

When the psychotherapist met Barry for the first time in 1993, he was 34 years old and single. He originally consulted her because of anxiety and depressive mood and Barry had had no prior psychiatric or psychotherapeutic experiences. Although he had known about his HIV diagnosis for nine years, he was still in the mild symptomatic phase. When their psychotherapeutic work terminated after two years, Barry was still healthy.

Barry is on AZT when the psychotherapeutic work is initiated. Somewhat later he enters a medical research project and AZT is terminated. However, his CD4 cell count decreases and he has to withdraw from the study. Barry perceives this as a punishment, but he doesn't know why, "It's just a feeling I have." His physician recommends him to start with AZT again, but Barry is skeptical, "That would mean, I guess, that I have AIDS." After some weeks he adheres to his physician's recommendation. As a result he gets in touch with HIV-related worries and feelings of being threatened but also persecuted by HIV, accompanied by grief and despair. On and off he feels death anxiety but there is also a longing for death. "I want to die because I don't want to suffer but I don't want to lose my life." He raises the question of how to go about the "impossible task to unite life with death." Another concern to Barry is his sense of not being acknowledged or seen by his parents, health personnel, and friends because of the infection. There are also fears of being rejected or abandoned by friends and potential partners because of HIV.

During the last semester of psychotherapy, Barry expresses fears of becoming sick and dying, "I don't want to die now." The fears evoke grief and psychic pain. "I'm so sad because my life will be so much shorter than others. And it is also so sad that I'll have to separate from my dearest and beloved ones." But there is also a lot of rage directed toward HIV. "It is so unfair. It is a punishment." The reason for being punished is that he, according to his own opinion, has been "promiscuous." When one of his friends dies of HIV disease it stirs up thoughts and feelings about his own death. He wants to be surrounded by friends "when I'm about to die." Further, he makes decisions related to all the practical aspects of his funeral. Eventually, Barry realizes in its existential sense that "the total separation" will come one day, when he will have to depart from and say good-bye to his beloved ones.

Richard

The second case vignette is the HIV scenario of Richard. He was in his early thirties and single when he started his psychotherapeutic work in 1987, which lasted six years. Earlier in this adult life, Richard had had some consultations with a psychiatrist and prior to his contact with the psychotherapist he had had seven months of therapeutic contact with a colleague of hers. The alleged reason for consulting the center was depressive mood and anxiety and he had known his HIV diagnosis for two years.

The psychotherapeutic work starts when Richard is in the mild symptomatic phase. He is then on HIV-related medication, which scares him and makes him very aware of HIV and the insight of "I cannot run away from HIV any more." From Richard's point of view, HIV is a punishment because he has been unfaithful.

The infection in combination with the treatment stirs up emotions of abandonment and vulnerability. Richard is dissatisfied with the way in which he is treated by the hospital staff, "They don't respect me and they make me sicker than I am." At other times he argues that "people are only interested in me because they feel sorry for me." He starts to take AZT evoking worries and fear of becoming sick and dying and he cries a lot when he gets in touch with these feelings. There are also fears related to becoming dependent and abandoned and Richard expresses that he wants to avoid these HIV-related thoughts and feelings. Symbolically, Richard describes HIV as a dragon on which he has put a leash by means of AZT. Ambivalent feelings toward AZT come to the forefront, "you know, to eat this poison the rest of your life and it is supposed to increase my quality of life—well, that's a bit weird."

At the beginning of the severe symptomatic phase Richard is "fed up with HIV." In contrast to his earlier attitude toward HIV as God's punishment, HIV is now viewed as a result of "my neurosis." Richard declares he wants to have access to a brand new HIV treatment but is not accepted because he does not fit the criteria. He gets angry and considers going abroad to try alternative medication. However, Richard does not carry through with these plans. Ironically he is diagnosed with CMV and then fits the inclusion criteria and starts with the medication. "Well, now I am in control of my treatment and myself." But his negative attitude toward the staff intensifies as Richard feels hurt and dehumanized by the hospital staff because "they don't listen to me and they don't believe in me." The medication initiates thoughts about his property, and his concerns related to life after death intensifies. He also starts questioning whether he should go on working. Richard's psychological well-being turns into psychic instability, and he finds the medication restricting his life. Once again, as Richard says, is he reminded of the reality of HIV. After terminating the treatment he recoups his psychological well-being.

Richard develops more symptoms and he reflects on the meaning of life and becomes more introverted, which is intensified when friends of his die. He asks himself how to leave his "footprints after death." When Richard's doctor informs him about a drastic CD4 cell drop, Richard strongly questions this information with an allegation to his "feeling well physically." Yet, he decides to write his will and to start to plan for his funeral with the feeling of "It's all so macabre." There is ambivalence toward the various treatment regimes, "It's good for my physical well-being but a disaster to my psychological well-being." Later Richard exclaims that "something is happening in my body" and he is terrified of developing brain damage (two years later on the same date he voices this concern, Richard dies). In parallel with physical deterioration and medication Richard expresses great worries, fears, sadness, and grief. Death anxiety and fear of abandonment are evoked, and he oscillates between despair and hope.

Richard becomes increasingly fatigued and wants to withdraw, "but my partner and friends do not respect me for that." At the same time he raises concerns about social death. His aggressive outbursts frighten him as he thinks they might be a manifestation of brain damage. Slowly Richard becomes aware that behind his aggressiveness and rage there is despair, grief, and death anxiety. His life space reduces, which is reinforced when he gets a port-a-cath. "It's negative because it's a reminder of HIV but practically it is positive." Richard is in and out of the hospital, and he becomes existentially aware of his impending death, which scares him. Along with more intensified medication and treatment he concludes, "My illusion about my immortality is broken and shattered into pieces. There is no way to run away from HIV."

Toward the end of this disease phase Richard's fearful attitude turns into a more positive one and his fighting spirit comes back. He is also more collected in his grief. "It is not as heavy as it was before and I want to make the best out of the rest of my life."

When Richard enters the terminal phase he is in a relatively good spirit despite his body deterioration. He stresses that he is not afraid of death any longer. As he gradually develops more symptoms he gets more worried about his health and his death anxiety comes back. Further he expresses his deep sadness and grief "that soon I'll have to separate from you all." Sometimes Richard feels like he is "a worthless package, which decays from the inside" and at other times he says "I have two sides; one is healthy and one is sick." After-death thoughts come to the surface and he is very much aware of his impending death, "I don't have that much time left, but I want to make the best of it." "My body is like a shell that is decayed and broken down. But behind this shell there is a healthy, fresh lemon and the lemon is my soul and I'm longing for the lemon to transform into a newborn baby and in that way my life experiences can be passed on." It is difficult for Richard to make up his mind whether he wants to be spread to the wind or to be buried in a coffin. His death anxiety comes and goes and so does despair and hope. Realizing he becomes more and more dependent upon others causes him great psychic pain and feelings of being hurt. Another salient emotion toward the end of his life is anger directed at medication and the hospital staff, in particular the physicians, "they don't keep me informed about my health status." Richard emphasizes his need to be in control and to have a frank and straightforward communication with the staff. He also feels increasingly alone but his lover is at his side and that comforts him tremendously. Richard becomes more and more exhausted, quite convinced "there is not much time left for me." He and his lover have decided to go to a spa and Richard is indeed anxious that he will not be able to make it. But he does and Richard dies the day after returning home.

Andy

When the psychotherapist met Andy for the first time in 1989, he had been diagnosed with HIV for two years and was in the asymptomatic phase. Andy was in his forties and single, and he consulted the therapist because of depressive mood and anxiety. He had earlier been in counseling. Our psychotherapeutic contact lasted three years.

In the asymptomatic phase HIV is not a topic except at one session, when Andy expresses his fear of being diagnosed with AIDS. In the third semester, Andy's health deteriorates quite rapidly, he is diagnosed with AIDS (six months after he expressed his AIDS concerns), and he enters the severe symptomatic phase. He discloses his HIV status to a friend and experiences "some relief."

Early on in the this disease phase Andy brings up his thoughts about having passive euthanasia "when the day comes, because I don't want to be on any life-support medication at that stage." He expresses his fear of disease progression and "for a moment" he gets in touch with death anxiety. Andy's progression fear is also reflected in his rumination of AIDS and he becomes preoccupied with his body and its signals, "something is happening in my body." Another theme is his thoughts about his funeral. Andy meets with a priest to discuss the arrangements. Eventually his progression fear subsides. However, Andy is aware of "time limitation" and brings up the subject of meaning in life. In the middle of the severe disease phase, Andy discloses his HIV status to his original family and friends, and he is well received.

The time awareness becomes more a focus as his health further deteriorates and he talks about "the count-down has started." Andy finds it difficult to take advantage of "the waiting," which he finds extremely taxing. He is from time to time working, although he is ambivalent toward whether he should continue to work. The ambivalence is also present as to his HIV medication as it is with respect to his longing to live versus his longing to die.

Andy starts to develop neurological symptoms and is hospitalized and he says "I've the sense that I don't have that much more time. I'm in the claws of HIV." His feelings of resignation are reflected in words such as, "I want to give in. I can't take it anymore. I want to terminate all treatment. I don't want to work anymore." However, Andy does not end the medication and he returns to work for some time. His health further deteriorates and Andy is upset that "everything in my life circles around that damn disease." His time concerns return and so do his death thoughts, which are manifested in suicidal ideation, "I want to be in control of death," as well as in his ambivalence toward death. Andy says "I want to live, but I want to escape my suffering. When death comes I want it to come quick." He also expresses his sadness in having to say good-byes.

Andy's health further deteriorates and he enters the terminal phase. He is sad and mourns that he has to die. "But I have given up. There is nothing to live for. I've reached the stage I've feared the most." He withdraws and becomes more introverted but appreciates having his family around him. The last time the psychotherapist meets Andy he says: "I've no worries, no anxiety, I'm just so tired." Andy dies the following day.

REFERENCES

1. Kübler-Ross E. *On Death and Dying*. London: Tavistock; 1970.
2. Hoffman MA. Counseling the HIV-infected client: A psychosocial model for assessment and intervention. *The Counseling Psychologist* 1991; 19(4):467–542.
3. Nilsson Schönnesson L. Traumatic and adaptation dimensions of HIV infection. In: Nilsson Schönnesson L., ed. *Sexual Transmission of HIV Infection. Risk Reduction, Trauma, and Adaptation*. New York: Haworth Press; 1992; 1–12.
4. Nilsson Schönnesson L. HIV infection: Trauma, psychic metabolism, and psychological well-being. A study of 29 gay HIV-positive men. Unpublished report (in Swedish). Stockholm; 1993.

9

The Shattered Self

WITH DR. KERSTIN FUGL-MEYER

As important as it is to recognize and appreciate the adaptation processes within the HIV disease scenario, it is as vital to acknowledge the internal psychological world through which these processes are mediated and can be understood. The internal psychological world refers here to the self, encompassing the individual's self-image and self-esteem. It constitutes the third component of the individual psychological landscape. The sense of self (or self-cohesion) provides the individual with a sense of stability. At first glance, these concepts may appear far away from HIV realities. However, we agree with Abramowitz and Cohen[1] that self psychology offers a useful psychodynamic bridge between the physical, social, and sexual consequences and the intrapsychic effects of HIV. The qualitative analysis of the psychotherapeutic notes of the 38 Swedish gay men supported this perspective in that we found a very large proportion of the psychotherapeutic work focused on the self. Further, just as HIV-related threats and psychological issues have to be processed and adapted to (Chapter 8), the men also struggled with processing and restoring their more or less shattered self. The latter is partly the result of the psychological impact of HIV on the individual's self. We would suggest that the HIV-disease adaptation processes interplay with the self adaptation processes and that they are both embedded in the existential context of death, freedom, isolation, and meaning.

In this chapter, we address, albeit in a preliminary way, the relevance and significance of the self and self adaptation processes in our understanding of the situation of being a gay man with HIV. As will be discussed in the first section, many gay men from early age on develop more or less poor self images, a sense of inadequacy, and a low self-esteem, that is, a vulnerable self. This is a result of among others psychological interpersonal difficulties during childhood and adolescence and social anti-gay attitudes and values (or homophobia) and their internalization.

In the second section, we argue that when the self is faced with the HIV infection, it easily becomes destabilized. By means of the qualitative analysis of the clinical notes, we identified the self as being compromised by psychological stressors. These were the wasting disease, mood distress, external and internal HIV persecutors, disrupted self needs (mirroring, twinship, and idealization), and activation of intimacy internal conflicts, self issues, and associations between HIV and parental images. Given that many gay men's vulnerable cohesive selfs antedate their HIV diagnosis, the self also becomes more susceptible to the attack of HIV.

We address in the third section the consequences of the psychological stressors on the self in terms of a shattered self. In the fourth section, we describe various means that the individual may make use of to adapt to the more or less shattered self.

In the fifth and final section of this chapter, we illuminate the interplay between the HIV disease scenarios and the self scenarios by means of two narratives from an interview study conducted by Nilsson Schönnesson[2] and three renarratizations based upon clinical vignettes.

SELF DEVELOPMENT OF GAY MEN

The Challenge in Developing a Cohesive Self

Generally speaking, gay men are faced with unique challenges in developing a cohesive sense of self[3] because of existing anti-gay attitudes and values in our Western heterosexual cultures. To be gay is still regarded with contempt and disgust by many people. There is no doubt that many gay men experience from an early age on rejection, abandonment, and lack of affirmation from the environment, including their original families.

In addition to love, every child needs to be mirrored, understood, accepted, and respected for who he is in terms of his thoughts, feelings, perceptions and their manifestations.[4] These needs have to be acknowledged and satisfied if a sound or an authentic self is to be developed. However, some parents are incapable of providing their child with this due to their own more or less severe psychological impairments. Some of the gay men in the psychotherapeutic material described a traumatic childhood by means of physical and psychological abuse, parental alcoholism, and longer or shorter time in an orphanage during their first years of life. Ours and others' clinical experience,[5,6] as well as nonclinical empirical studies,[7] indicate that some gay men may recall their father as being distant or nonemotional toward them during childhood. Others may describe their father as being present but uninvolved in the family, controlling, or unpredictable. When this was the case, some men expressed their longing for a father image, as exemplified by Norman's experiences. He perceived his father as never being there for him during his childhood, which Norman regretted tremendously. He dealt with his grief by writing a novel, in which he was the father of a son. The father was the kind of father that Norman had always longed for as a child. By means of this novel, Norman was able to work through his grief over a father who was never there for him. Mothers were, within the psychotherapeutic notes, usually depicted as "a divine mother," "nonauthentic," "nonalive," "engulfing," "incestuous," and "boundless." Whereas some men experienced that their mother did not "allow" the father into the dyad of the mother-son, "she kept him away from me," others reported their sense of not being protected from the mother by the father. Over one-half of the men (59%) reflected upon their experiences of and disappointments in not having had "good enough" parents during their upbringing. To some of them, the psychotherapist in the course of the psychotherapeutic work was perceived as a new parental figure, which also caused psychological pain. Gerald reflects:

> Your way of treating me makes me aware that parents don't need to be the way mine were. But it also hurts to become aware of this, because now I realize how much I have been missing during my upbringing.

A recurring theme among some of the men was the experience that they had to satisfy the needs of one or both of the parents, whereas their own needs and wishes were of a second order. They described feelings of being rejected or not affirmed by the parents. There are also parents who punish or strongly object to their child when he behaves or expresses thoughts that are "deviant" from their value systems and norms. It was for example quite common that some gay men remembered feelings of being "different" or being an "outsider" during their childhood and adolescence. This "outsider" status manifested itself in various ways but a quite common one is "atypical" gender roles. Isay[5] argues that the paternal withdrawal is the result of the father's awareness that the son does not act as other boys or their son is too closely attached to the father for his own comfort. Some gay men have also experienced rejection or humiliation as a "weakling" from their peers in their childhood because of "atypical" behavior and manners. Others described that peers had mobbed them because of being overweight. Later the gay man may infer his "outsider" status in childhood as the first sign of his gayness. As Jeffrey says, "I remember that I was mobbed at school but I really never understood why. But maybe my peers had figured out my homosexuality before I did."

As the child is dependent upon his parents and their love and concerns the child does what it takes to get their appreciation. The child may for example adapt more or less completely to the parents' needs and wishes, which may lead to a "false self."[8] This is an attitude in which the individual behaves and thinks in a way that satisfies the parent(s) (or others) needs rather than his own. His authentic self cannot or is not allowed to be experienced. Andrew explains:

> You know, there wasn't really any room for me in our family. I realize now that my needs have never been taken seriously. My parents put me on a pedestal. They saw me as an adult and if I had fallen down they would have punished me. When I was sad my parents reinterpreted that as me being tired and I needed to sleep. I should be there for my father to satisfy his psychological needs. My role has always been to be there for others and in that way I have received love. When I try to show who I really am, my family rejects me.

> However, when I put on a mask, well then they approve of me. I strongly feel that no one likes or loves me the way I am in the bottom of my heart. I am so very much longing for my inner, bright rooms in which I can find peace and harmony and find something divine where my own needs will take precedence. What has taken place on my internal scene has never been allowed to be expressed but has been adapted to the formalities of life. The only way to express the inner scene has been through music.

Another possibility to the child is to split off certain aspects of the self that are disliked by or displeasing to the parent(s). The child attempts to maintain a self that he believes his parents find acceptable and loveable. He learns that compliance to their expectations and wishes is rewarded with acceptance and love. But compliance has its price; to give up parts of the authenticity of the self leads to the development of a "mask of niceness." It can take on an indiscriminate character. The goal of the "mask of niceness" is to avoid being disliked and the secondary goal is to be liked. The dynamics of both the false self and the mask of niceness is self-deception "in order to gain the acceptance and approval of others"[9] (p. 34). When the self is not fully authentic, it also becomes quite vulnerable. The gay man thus runs the risk of developing in his early years a vulnerable self.

Societal Anti-Gay Attitudes

Given the heterosexual culture, it is not an overstatement in saying that the solidification of the self is significantly more difficult for the gay than the heterosexual man. Ericson[10] underscores that one important component of the psychological development is that the child/adolescent interact with people and activities of his stream of society that confirm his self. Whereas heterosexual adolescents are directly and indirectly supported and confirmed in various ways in his heterosexual identity process, the gay adolescent is not. "Indeed, there are no rituals, activities, or rites of passage that confirm a gay man's identity"[9] (p. 28).

Another important factor in the individual's self development is, according to Sullivan,[11] the appraisals of others. These appraisals can both facilitate and cause difficulties in psychological growth. Because of the anti-gay attitudes in our society, gay men anticipate negative reactions when they disclose their gay identity. Too often, the feared anticipation turns into reality in that the man is met with contempt, rejection, and detachment when he discloses his gay identity. In contrast to the heterosexual men who from early on is told that his identity is "good" and "normal," the gay man is directly and indirectly told that his identity is "bad," "abnormal," "sinful," "perverse," and "pathological." Thus, he is stigmatized as a result of the anti-gay value system. Stigmatization refers to devaluation and dehumanization of the person based on his same gender preference as such. In other words, his whole self is "bad," "disturbed," or "not good enough."

Internalized Anti-Gay Attitudes

Not only is the gay man exposed to external but also to internal anti-gay attitudes and stigmatization. These could also be referred to as external and internal anti-gay persecutors. The latter refers to what the individual within a negative societal context incorporates and internalizes the societal negativism (i.e., internalized homophobia). Consequently, he develops a more or less harsh self-contempt and even self-hatred. Isay argues that it is not gayness as such that is despised by gay men but "what they have been taught as children to perceive as being different" and what has been labeled as being "feminine"[5] (p. 129). The internalized anti-gay attitudes are thus super-imposed on an already vulnerable self. Therefore, the individual's self-esteem, self-image, and self-cohesion run the risk to be further affected in a negative direction and he may feel injured, worthless, undesirable, and unlovable, and perceive his sexuality as disgusting.

Kertzner argues that the overriding developmental task of gay men during adulthood is to maintain a positive sense of the self in "an assumptive world that negates their existence and which directly or indirectly rewards their invisibility and punishes healthy disclosure" (Brooks cited in Kertzner,[12] p. 90). Taking these external and internal anti-gay persecutors together, we may ask how it is that anyone who experiences them "for a lifetime can manage not to have a feeling of loss of self, of false self"[13] (p. 270).

Cornett[9] makes an interesting observation in discussing differences between rejections faced by gay men and other racial or minority groups.

> There is one vast difference.... Members of racial and ethnic groups that face hatred and rejection on that basis can be virtually assured of not being rejected within their own families. Gay men have no such guarantee and the majority of gay men face some emotional or physical rejection when they assert their identities to their families.[9] (p. 31)

"Solutions" of External and Internal Anti-Gay Persecutors

In order to psychologically survive the external and internal anti-gay persecutors and to protect his vulnerable self from further attacks, the individual tries to find solutions. One available "solution" is to completely split off and deny one's same gender preference and in that way the false self is also reinforced. Heterosexual marriage can be one form of this denial. Some may want to change their sexuality. Others decide to hide their gayness to the nongay world, which leads to living a double life. Still another "solution" is to try to compensate for one's "badness" (i.e., one's gayness) by striving for impeccability in one's appearance, work, home, and so forth, that is, "the impeccable mask." Kenneth phrased it in a symbolic way: "No one is going, and I really mean no one, is going to have a chance to accuse me for having creased clothes."

All these "solutions" may impede the integration of a sound gay identity.[14] However, it has to be remembered that there are indeed gay men who have developed a positive and cohesive self and gay identity. Nevertheless, it is our impression that also among these men there are rudiments of internalized anti-gay persecutors that under certain stressors (like the HIV infection) may be reactivated.

PSYCHOLOGICAL STRESSORS

The self—and to many gay men their vulnerable self—is further attacked by the HIV disease. The qualitative analysis unfolded seven psychological stressors that assaulted the gay men's self: a wasting disease, mood distress, external and internal HIV persecutors, disrupted self needs, an activation of intimacy internal conflicts, self issues, and associations between HIV and parental images. Although we describe each of them separately, the psychological stressors may interact with one another.

The Wasting Disease

As described in Chapter 4 the body is an integral part of the self. Thus, when HIV attacks the body immune system it also assails the individual's psychological immune system, that is, the self, which has a psychological life-giving function. The intrapsychic relationship between the physical body and the psychological self is termed the body self.[15] Consequently "a subjective experience of defectiveness through disfigurement or malfunctioning of the body is destabilizing to self-organization"[1] (p. 207).

HIV disease like other chronic or terminal diseases shakes earlier taken-for-granted assumptions about possessing a smoothly functioning body[16] and disrupts a sense of wholeness of body and self. As long as the person does not experience the body effects on a daily level or can control those effects or when other concerns take precedence, he usually ignores or minimizes the disease.[16] He can objectify and keep the HIV infection and his body at the margin of his self, thus preserving the sense of a body self unity he had prior to the diagnosis. Yet, in the face of the HIV disease progression, people often experience various modes of living with the disease at different times. When the person notes physical changes and diminished bodily functions, he experiences an altered body.[16] The person with HIV is repeatedly challenged with destabilization of the body self as he experiences new bodily losses. The body may feel alien and the person may experience the feeling that HIV controls him, "I'm in the claws of HIV," and the body self is more or less disrupted. To some men it is as if the body disease has been translated into HIV within his self, as "I am HIV." The past body becomes the yardstick against which he compares his altered body. Simon describes his current life situation (in the severe symptomatic disease phase) in terms of "two pictures." One of the pictures is bigger than the other. The bigger one represents Simon's "well-known, familiar grounds. There I could do all wonderful things and there were no limits or boundaries in my life." The smaller one symbolizes his current situation, which is quite new to him.

> I'm struggling to get accustomed to this new picture frame and it is so difficult and painful. You know, I don't have the energy to go swimming three times a week as I used to for example.

To some this "new, smaller picture frame" may be such a blow to the self, that the person refuses to try to do anything that he enjoyed before he developed severe symptoms. William for example expresses his attitude: "No, I'm not going to go bicycling because if I'm not able to ride the same distance as before, well forget it."

Others may view HIV disease as an enemy with whom they must battle. The body self is destabilized but they struggle to keep up with their prediagnostic body self unity. It is extremely hard for them to face, albeit to accept, more restricted lives. The person may also reconcile himself to the HIV disease for years. He acknowledges and tolerates the disease within limits but he does not accept it. Still others struggle to keep their bodies functioning and therefore to keep their lives as "normal" as possible. They objectify their body to a lesser extent, cease to compare their body against "the past yardstick," and integrate new body facts into their lives. The ill body becomes familiar and the person begins to live with it and to unify body and self again. Because of reoccurring HIV-related symptoms, the "body familiarity" is, however, not a fixed but a temporary state that may last for longer or shorter periods. During the "latency" people may adapt to the disease for the time being at least. However, there are also people who never adapt to bodily impairment. Adapting, according to Charmaz, refers to altering life and self to accommodate to physical losses and to reunify body and self and living with illness without living solely for it. The illness is viewed as an integral part of self. "Thus, chronically ill people who move beyond loss and transcend stigmatizing negative labels define themselves as much more than their bodies and as much more than an illness"[16] (p. 660). Mark Kidel quoted in Charmaz, advocates "reclaiming our illnesses as expressions of our own being" to gain authenticity[17] (p. 672).

Mood Distress

As shown in Chapter 5, the psychological issues accompanying the HIV disease are experienced in different ways by the men and across the disease phases. Likewise, gay men living with HIV are not a homogenous group either with respect to the impact of HIV-related threats and psychological issues on their psychological functioning or with regard to psychological functioning over the disease phases (Chapter 6).

Bearing in mind the drama of the HIV disease scenario and all of its adaptational tasks and challenges, it is not surprising that gay men with HIV may at least sometime experience an imbalance between the burdens and their available resources. Many of the men in Dr. Schönnesson's case load had reached the peak of imbalance, and they therefore sought professional help. They had reached a "dead end"[18] and the men described feelings of hopelessness, negative resignation, existing but not living, and being stuck in the HIV trauma and its mourning. Such a "dead end" mode of living may contribute to destabilizing the self.

External and Internal HIV Persecutors

A third psychological stressor on the self is the potential external and internal HIV persecutors. The former ones refer to the potential stigmatizing and rejecting environment. But the individual may also become his own, internal, persecutor. Just as the individual internalizes the societal anti-gay attitudes, he may also internalize the negative societal attitudes toward HIV and thus they become a more or less integral part of the individual's self. The negative HIV image haunts the individual in terms of psychological persecutors such as guilt, shame, self-blame, degradation, and devaluation. The individual may also perceive feelings of, among others, anxiety, helplessness, powerlessness, and hopelessness as persecutors. Both the external and internal HIV-related persecutors thus threaten the self with destabilization.

Disrupted Self Needs

The necessity of having mirroring, twinship, and idealizing needs met in the development and maintenance of the self and self-esteem was discussed in Chapter 4. Mirroring refers to our need for affirmation and recognition of others. Twinship needs contain the experience of feeling an essential alikeness with others, and idealizing describes the experience of being soothed, protected, and accepted by an admired and respected person. These needs may be disrupted by the stigma associated with HIV and loss of friends,[1] and the negative HIV image. For example, rejection or abandonment by lovers, family, friends, colleagues, who have served important mirroring and twinship functions, may deprive the person of the mirroring that he needs so badly in the situation of having HIV. The clinical data showed that almost one-half of the gay men in the terminal phase and one-third in the mild symptomatic phase reported having these experiences. Multiple losses of friends and the disappearance of social networks, as experienced by almost one-half of the men in the mild symptomatic disease phase, also disrupted the mirroring as well as the twinship functions of gay subcultures. When the gay man with HIV in relation to gay subculture(s) experiences feelings of being different as to serostatus he may perceive that his twinship bonds to the subculture are disconnected. When a beloved person dies who had provided the individual with psychological protection and soothing at rough times, the idealizing needs of the living person are heavily circumscribed. As the disease progresses, the person's idealizing needs become more salient. He yearns for protection, calmness, and safety. When they are not met, the individual experiences disappointment, which can undermine his self-cohesion. As described in Chapter 5, disappointment can be expressed through aggressive outbursts, often directed at health care staff, in particular the physicians. However, underneath aggressiveness and disappointment there are feelings of helplessness and hopelessness.

The most fundamental route for fulfilling mirroring, twinship, and idealizing needs is sexual contact. To most gay men sexuality is, as has been emphasized earlier, a vital component of their self. Sexuality provides them with support and confirmation of worth. Some of the men in the clinical material were themselves indeed conscious about and expressed clearly that they used sex as a way to be confirmed. When diagnosed with HIV this important "avenue for mirroring" is interrupted. Along the disease progression, the sexual mirroring disruption becomes even more prominent. Abramowitz and Cohen make a very important remark in discussing HIV prevention among gay men with HIV. If for example unprotected anal sex stabilized the self with soothing and merging or unprotected oral sex provided a sense of affirmation,

> then the extent that self-stability is threatened by abandonment of these unsafe sex practices, the gay man will resist safer sex alternatives. The specific selfobject needs met by the unsafe practices must first be emphatically analyzed before safer sex alternatives can be found that also meet those needs.[1] (p. 214)

Activation of Intimacy Internal Conflicts, Self Issues, and Associations between HIV and Parental Images

The qualitative analysis of the psychotherapeutic notes showed that the HIV disease appeared to function as a "radar" of psychological conflicts, in particular in relation to intimacy, and self issues in terms of mirroring needs. Further, the analysis revealed that the virus might represent parental images.

Yet, given the intrusiveness of the HIV infection into the physical as well as the psychological immune system, we do not think it is a coincidence that these issues were brought to the surface among the gay men. In Chapter 4, we described the fear of psychological death in terms of physical threats and here we find that specific psychological stressors induce the fear of psychological death. This is illustrated below in that the internal intimacy conflicts, mirroring needs, and parental images are all colored by the fear of psychological death.

Internal Intimacy Conflicts

Intimacy is about closeness to another person and results "when an outsider is allowed.... into the person's concept of self—a potentially threatening thing—creating an acceptable feeling of vulnerability"[19] (p. 207). Another way to put it is to dare to merge with another person without being fearful of losing oneself, but to maintain one's separateness. Isay emphasizes that "the capacity to fall in love and to maintain a relationship over time requires a high degree of self-esteem or 'healthy narcissism' "[5] (p. 92). He also argues that many gay men are "angry, hurt, and reluctant to risk the possibility of further rejection or to expose a partner with the rage which they perceive within themselves"[5] (p. 85).

The vast majority of the gay men in this study, most of them single, brought up intimacy problems, in particular in the first two disease phases. These internal intimacy conflicts, however, antedated the HIV diagnosis. Tom, to whom intimacy difficulties were a core theme of the therapy, asked himself whether he would have been HIV negative today if he had been into therapy many years ago. "Maybe then I wouldn't have had that much sex but would have dared to get involved emotionally with another guy."

Given the potential vulnerable self and poor self-esteem of gay men, it is not surprising to find an ambivalent stance toward intimacy. On the one hand, there is a longing for intimacy and on the other hand, there is anxiety associated with entering a love relationship. Some dread that every relationship will end up in disaster. Others raise the question, "Why do I always choose the wrong type of guy?" These men talked about intimacy fear in terms of dependency, coming too close, intrusion, engulfment, rejection, and abandonment. The psychological denominator of these fears is a fear of psychological death—to become no one.

Some of the men who were currently in a love relationship also talked about their fear of becoming or being too dependent upon their partner, or to be or to become "trapped" in the relationship. Fear of abandonment also appeared. A few of them were in a relationship that they found abusive and humiliating, but they stayed because, as Frank notes:

> One has to appreciate that someone wants you. And it's better to stay than to leave—one never knows if there will be someone else out there for you.

On the other hand, it is also plausible that staying in a destructive relationship is a way to avoid intimacy.

One aspect of intimacy is sexuality. One-half of the gay men in this study reported that their sexual interest or desire had decreased or vanished completely. Most of these men were in the asymptomatic or mild symptomatic phase. Most of those men who were engaged in a love relationship, in which there were intimacy problems, also described a decline in their sexual interest or desire. The analysis further showed that some of the single men had feelings of guilt or shame related to sexuality or had great difficulties in merging sex and love. About one-third of them linked their sexual "abstinence" to fear of intimacy, whereas a few others regarded sex as a protection against intimacy.

Self Issues

Current mirroring needs were a salient theme among the men as reflected in words such as, "I want to be seen as a whole person." This wish is in sharp contrast to some men's experience of their physician "who only regards me as a virus. I am only of interest to him as long as I can provide him with symptoms." This example also illustrates how the person can become a jealous part in the triangulation of patient, doctor, and the disease. He feels excluded and ignored, and not treated for his own sake; the disease is the center of attention. Others emphasize their desire to be "confirmed/acknowledged." However, the salience of mirroring needs varied depending upon the disease phase. One-half and one-third of the men in the mild symptomatic and asymptomatic phases respectively talked about these concerns. In the severe disease phase, only a small minority expressed the theme of mirroring, and in the terminal phase there was none.

Almost one-half of the men reflected over the lack of parental mirroring during their childhood of whom almost all also expressed current mirroring needs. It is quite plausible that the HIV disease in these men reactivated an earlier inadequate mirroring milieu.

As the self needs are of such vital importance in sustaining self-esteem and a sense of self, the lack or disruption of having, for example, the mirroring needs met may lead to a sense of being no one, that is, psychological death.

Parental Images

The HIV disease may evoke associations between the virus and parental images. Roger for example experienced the HIV infection as being just as intrusive as his mother. He had fantasies that HIV would catch up with him (i.e., he would become sick), if he in any way was assertive toward his mother.

> They both want to be in charge of my life. It is like I don't have the right to live my own life. It is like they both want to kill me if I don't follow their guidelines.

In other cases, the man talked about his partner or the parent in such a way that the therapist shared with him her associations of the psychological similarities between the partner/parent and the virus. The client in general validated such associations. Nicholas for example perceived his boyfriend and their relationship as "suffocating." To others, HIV represented their alcoholic father. Both the disease and the father were perceived as unpredictable, frightening, and threatening. It also happens that the psychotherapist becomes the symbolic representation of HIV; she or he is perceived as "dangerous" or "threatening" in that she inflicts the client with pain and suffering.

THE SHATTERED SELF

The vulnerability to the psychological stressors differs between people and may change over time, and so does their impact on the self. The ways in which individuals perceive, approach, and adapt to the psychological stressors depend on a variety of psychological, cognitive, and social factors. Although we do not discuss or provide clinical data on personality structures in this book, we still want to make the point that the degree to which the personality is integrated and well functioning does play a role in the adaptation process. Gay men in general,[5,20] as well as those with HIV, represent a personality spectrum from those with a structured, cohesive personality with adaptive defense mechanisms to those with a more or less chaotic, unstructured, poorly integrated personality with less adaptive defenses. Those men who are characterized by a less well-integrated personality are more vulnerable to stressors, which in turn impedes their adaptation process.

The individual's life history, current life context, as well as his cognitive and social tools are other factors that influence the adaptation process. As a result of the adaptation process, the individual's self is more or less shattered. The qualitative analysis revealed that the gay men's self oscillated between a shattered and a restored self over time. In other words, neither the shattered nor the restored self is a static phenomenon, but the self is taken on an odyssey. This process is illuminated in the three renarratives that are presented later in the chapter. The clinical data showed that at times, there was a direct link between HIV-related physical and sexual stressors and a reshattered self as manifested in feelings of, among others, being hurt, violated, unloveable, not good enough, unworthy, and internally empty.

Dr. Schönnesson's psychotherapeutic notes indicated that the shattered self of the men could be described in terms of a vulnerable self, a devalued self-image, and dualism. These three aspects of the shattered self are, however, not independent but interdependent of one another. For example, a person who devalues himself or vacillates in his self-perception as a little boy/grown-up contributes to a vulnerable self.

The Vulnerable Self

Two-thirds of the gay men in the asymptomatic phase pondered about their vulnerable self, and the equivalent number in the mild and severe symptomatic phases was over one-half. None of the men who were in the terminal phase, however, talked about a vulnerable self. Regardless of disease phase, the vulnerable self was usually depicted in terms like a sense of emptiness, rootless, no internal substance, chaos, insecurity, and difficulties to set or to maintain boundaries with others. Some men also expressed boredom, little empathy with themselves, and contempt for one's own feelings. These could be interpreted as manifestations of a vulnerable self, just as their mirroring needs could be. It is most likely that the men had been struggling with the vulnerable self before HIV, but it is further challenged and reinforced by the HV disease.

One consequence of a shattered self is often a sense of having lost control "or direction over my life." As control is a psychological defense, the need to regain control is thus of vital concern. In order to do so, however, it takes a restored self. The significance of the need to be in control is shown in the clinical material. The vast majority of the men in the asymptomatic phase, in which over two-thirds described a vulnerable self, talked explicitly about their need to be in control, to regain a defense mechanism. Yet, because of the defensive character of control, the men could not exemplify which ways to achieve control.

Devalued Self-Image

About one-third of the gay men talked about themselves in humiliating terms, such as having no value, not being good enough, being a failure, worthless, and a second-class citizen. The feelings of those men who described themselves as having low self-respect or self-confidence are usually the consequence of self-devaluation. Some of the men related explicitly their devalued self image to their HIV disease or gayness whereas others did not—at least not consciously.

Dualism

The dualistic aspect of the shattered self, which is most prominent in the mild symptomatic phase, is manifested in dual self-perceptions and good/bad. The dual self-perceptions and the good/bad aspects refer, within this context, to evaluative judgments of oneself, which cause the individual psychological pain. The dual self-perception is manifested in descriptions of oneself as hedonistic versus dutiful, false versus authentic, introvert versus extrovert, child versus grown-up, emotionally warm versus cold, sex love versus sex hate.

In the good/bad dimension, the gay man portrays himself as "bad." In the individual's fantasy, the "bad" part of him is filled with aggression or rage, which is a potential danger to others. This aggressive potential is frightening to the individual. Charles notes:

> If I would let go of all my aggression I would become a ruthless person and there would be an anarchy within me. The bad part of me would be able to kill everything.

The partner or the psychotherapist designates the "good" dimension. One possible psychodynamic interpretation of the good/bad dimension would be that the "bad" part of him represents the HIV infection. Within the individual, on an unconscious level, there is a fear of his "bad"/HIV part intruding, hurting, or even killing the "good," that is, the partner or the psychotherapist. Medication may also be perceived as good/bad.

We find it psychologically noteworthy that the dualistic aspect of the shattered self is most salient in the mild symptomatic phase. Entering this phase it becomes harder to deny HIV, and as shown in Chapter 4, the physical threats were perceived in terms of bewilderment. Thus, it could be argued that what is happening in the HIV disease scenario—physical awareness of the disease and psychological bewilderment as to sick/healthy roles—is transformed into the self scenario. The individual becomes aware of the psychologically contrary dimensions of his self and he experiences bewilderment.

THE SHATTERED SELF ADAPTATION PROCESSES

The individual needs to restore a more or less shattered self to achieve a more cohesive self. A stabilized self is also crucial to facilitate the approach and adaptation to the spectrum of HIV-related physical, social, sexual threats, and psychological issues. Dr. Schönnesson's clinical experience is, however, that at the bottom line the vast majority of the gay men were not only yearning for a restored self, but even more so for a stronger authentic self.

But as we have pointed out earlier, the HIV-related threats, psychological issues, and the psychological stressors of the self are of a reoccurring character, which of course influences the stability of the self. In other words, the self adaptation processes, like the HIV-disease ones, should be viewed as a spiral model rather than as a stage model.

The individual who experiences a shattered self may use different approaches in his attempt to restore it. The qualitative analysis revealed that the gay men mainly used the mirroring, twinship, and idealizing approaches in relation to their social network and the psychotherapeutic relationship.

The Social Network Approach

Some of the gay men explained very specifically that they needed to be confirmed and seen by others to feel like "a whole person." Others were actively engaged in the Body Positive group, which provided them with twinship bonds. Besides, it is quite likely that being part of the Body Positive group may help the person to face separation and to mourn losses; the organization becomes a symbol of separation and togetherness. The commitment also granted them with confirmation of worth and improvement in self-esteem, just as adopting the role of HIV informant did. In this way the men could "transform a personal ordeal into something of value for others and for themselves"[1] (p. 216).

A few of the men established a connection to spirituality or another Christian denomination, which met the individual's idealizing needs. The commitment to the Body Positive group may be another example whereby the individual feels protected and soothed.

The Psychotherapeutic Approach

The mirroring and idealizing needs can also be met through the relationship to the psychotherapist. When the client experiences that he is free to express his fears and concerns, without being rejected, abandoned, or ridiculed, and that the therapist can recognize and mirror these feelings, the client encounters the therapist to be "good" and that there is an attachment between the two of them. This sense of emotional freedom can facilitate the restoration of the self.[21] The attachment, including trust and intimacy, between client and therapist is often referred to as dependency or idealization.

The qualitative analysis of the psychotherapeutic notes showed that along the disease phases more of the gay men expressed their attachment to the therapist (39% in phase 1, 62% in phase 2, 63% in phase 3, and 77% in phase 4). The attachment was reflected in words like "I trust you," "Promise that you won't abandon me," "I've missed you," "I'm so happy to see you again, but I don't know why," "I'm always looking forward to our sessions." In the severe or the terminal phases some men expressed their need of the therapist as, "When I'm getting worse I want you to come more often because I feel so safe with you." Others expressed their wish to have the psychotherapist in the room when he was dying. Still others extended the attachment even after death by asking the therapist to read a poem (chosen by themselves) or to say some words about him at his funeral.

Attachment and its concomitant feelings of ambivalence are expected to develop in any psychotherapeutic relationships. However, among people with HIV the psychological ramifications of the HIV disease color the attachment. From a psychodynamic perspective, HIV (like cancer) often represents, consciously and unconsciously, the "bad" part of the individual's self. The disease is also perceived as an internal intruder or persecutor. Both the "bad" and the persecutory aspects of HIV contribute to a shattered self. In the individual's struggle to restore his self, the psychotherapist becomes an important person in that she or he usually represents "good" and "health." Quite a few of the gay men made comments like: "There is no question in my mind but you are healthy," or "You just can't be sick," or "I would never forgive you if you got sick."

However, the attachment to the therapist usually evokes anxiety, as closeness further threatens the person's psychological integrity and independence. The integrity has already been attacked by HIV, and as the disease progresses into the severe symptomatic and terminal phases, the individual's independence is heavily circumscribed. The closeness to the therapist may also evoke the symbolic representation of the therapist as HIV. Consequently, the therapeutic relationship becomes colored by ambivalence. The individual tries to find various "solutions" to the ambivalence. One is to deny attachment by rejecting the therapist as a way to ward off fears of being rejected by her or him. Another solution is to try to keep an inner distance to the therapist and thus to preserve a sense of autonomy. In the analysis of the psychotherapeutic notes, we found two conditions that could be interpreted as examples of the inner distance. The first condition is when the client "forgets" the contents between the sessions. The other one is when the client makes "temporary breaks" in the therapeutic work but always makes sure that he is welcome back when he needs to. These breaks could be interpreted as the client's "internal adaptation clock," the client's way to fulfill his need of internal distance to the therapist. Another interpretation would be, following Langs,[22] that attachment or psychotherapeutic frames may trigger death anxiety, and thus the client needs to modulate the psychotherapeutic context. The ambivalent feelings toward the therapeutic relationship is well captured in Philip's comment: "You are an unpleasant pleasure."

The mirroring and idealizing needs can be worked through by means of transference. Discussions and struggles over the concept of transference, its definition, and operationalization have been going on for years within the psychotherapeutic communities. We refer here to transference as an interpersonal, compensatory process in which the client uses the psychotherapist to stabilize his self and to achieve a wholeness of his self.[9,14] Thus, the therapist compensates for the client's deficits in his mirroring and idealizing (but also twinship) needs. In the mirroring transference, the therapist needs to explore and acknowledge the devalued self of the client, work these through, and actively affirm the self.

The idealized transference stems from the client's wish to get unconditioned love, total security, and absolute trust, that is, to be protected. The client invests his idealized needs into the therapeutic relationship to fulfill them. As the disease progresses the person with HIV realizes that the therapist cannot protect him from HIV, which evokes an understandable disappointment in him. It is important that the therapist acknowledges the disappointment and together with the client works it through. By remaining caring and present, the therapist most often can restore the disrupted idealization. The transference usually intensifies in the terminal phase. Dreifuss-Kattan[21] equates the idealized transference with "the primary partnership," that is, the relationship between the child and his mother. Nevertheless, this "primary relationship" is always threatened by impending loss and thus has to be cared for at all times. Consequently, the relationship also has an ambivalent character. It is manifested in the wish to withdraw so as to anticipate separation on the one hand, and to cling so as to avoid separation on the other hand.

Manifestations of a Restored Self

A restored self can be manifested in many ways. The gay men did not use the concept of a restored self but used other words, which we interpret as its reflections. The most common words being used are resilience, psychological well-being, a positive self-image, improved self-esteem and self-confidence, more sensitive to one's own needs, and able to set boundaries with others. Most often, the men used a combination of these words. From our point of view, these words indirectly reflect an increased sense of control, choice, vitality, and self-respect.

CASE STUDIES AND CLINICAL VIGNETTES

In this section we first present two case studies, based on an interview study[2] conducted by Dr. Schönnesson, that highlight two different self scenarios and adaptation processes of the HIV diagnosis. Second, three renarratives are offered to illuminate the interplay between the HIV disease scenario and the self scenario as well as their adaptational processes.

Case Studies

George

George, a self-identified gay man, is 39 years old. He would like to live as a heterosexual "just because it would make life much easier." George's parents, who are dead, never learned about his gayness. In 1986, George got his HIV diagnosis. He is a teacher and he likes his job a lot. However, he often runs into conflicts with his colleagues and George feels abandoned and stigmatized at work. He has during his entire adulthood always lived on his own and never been involved in a steady partner relationship. However, over the years, according to George, he has had thousands of sex partners but no steady relationship. George's present social network is almost nonexistent. He used to socialize somewhat with a small group of gay men pre-HIV but today it very rarely happens. He does not feel liked and appreciated by others, and George detaches himself from others and grows more and more isolated. This social withdrawal attitude, according to George, has always been there but has become more profound after the HIV diagnosis.

George and his two siblings were brought up in an abusive family. His father was an alcoholic and physically abused his wife and children and George was very afraid of him: "You know, he was so unpredictable. He was a bad guy." He describes his mother in a very positive way: "She was a darling and very affectionate.

Thanks to her I did not go crazy." But it is highly likely that the positive relationship to his mother has not been able to compensate for the bad father figure. So as a result, George's childhood experiences and conditions have contributed to his negative self-image and low self-esteem. Another result of his upbringing is his mistrust in other people, viewing the world as hostile and himself as socially incompetent and unable to remain in a long-term relationship. George finds some consolation in being outdoors in nature but most of all his consolation is the liquor bottle. He drinks almost every day after work.

George feels "scared to death" and anxiety-ridden by his infection. He sees himself as a victim, totally engulfed by HIV, with a total lack of sense of mastery. George also reports feelings of shame and self blame for being HIV seropositive. He experiences HIV-related intrusive thoughts and feelings as well as strong emotional AIDS rumination stress, and he is very afraid of becoming sick. George assesses the risk of becoming sick as high, and he tries to avoid these distressful thoughts and feelings but without any real success. A couple of persons within George's social network know about his HIV status. He has decided to commit suicide the day he gets the first symptoms: "I don't want any of my relatives to see a tragic case." George gives the following description of his life after being diagnosed with HIV: "It is like a big, deep, black hole."

George's internal world is characterized by its negative, hostile, and persecuting atmosphere with the exception of his positive mother figure. Here we can see an internal persecuting scenario in which George finds himself completely left out. He feels persecuted not only by the HIV infection but also by the external world, regardless of HIV. The fear of being abandoned and extinguished is there more or less constantly, and George feels that there is really no one in his world to trust. But he expresses a longing for help, care, and support in coping with the hostile internal and external worlds.

George's internal resources appear to be reduced due to his negative self-image and his fragile self-esteem. That leads to difficulties in providing a protective shelter from AIDS depressive ruminations and death anxiety. He starts drinking when anxiety and the demons intrude on him. In addition to free-floating anxiety, George also reports psychosomatic and depressive symptoms.

Within George's internal world, we can see a parallel between his experiences with his father and with the HIV infection. Both represent the evil/bad, the unpredictable and uncertainty and they threaten him with separation and annihilation. The HIV infection reactivates his traumatic childhood experiences with his father, which involved anxiety and feelings of powerlessness and helplessness. George tries to avoid HIV-related confrontations, intrapsychic conflict, and anxiety by means of an avoidant coping attitude including heavy drinking. But his worries, concerns, and stress often become too powerful, and he enters a vicious circle. To look for help, support, and consolation in others is not easy for George as he fears relationship catastrophes (i.e., to be disappointed or abandoned) when turning to other persons. On the other hand, by withdrawing socially, George is not mirrored by others, and he becomes alone with and vulnerable to the HIV persecutor and all its related feelings of psychological suffering and anxiety. Since George does not have access to "good enough" internal resources, it becomes difficult for him to handle the HIV situation. He becomes, in other words, alone with the HIV persecutor since he does not dare to seek help, support, and care from others since that would reactivate his anxieties related to abandonment and annihilation. To summarize, George is just as fearful of life as of death and from that perspective we can understand the reason for George turning to liquor and temporarily finding a protective shelter toward his miserable life situation.

Andrew

Andrew is 23 years old with no steady partner. He has no professional training but has made his living through various unskilled jobs. In 1987, Andrew was notified about his HIV seropositivity and since then, he has from time to time been on sick leave due to psychological stress. Andrew is ashamed of his gayness and his, as he claims, "immoral sexual life." He expresses wishes that he "should have waited for the right man." Andrew describes that he has many casual sexual encounters and acquaintances. He stresses his longing for finding trust and security in a father figure. Andrew expresses some mistrust toward others, but at the same time, he is eager to seek help and support in others. It is, however, difficult for Andrew to remain within an intimate relationship. There is only one man (who works within the HIV field) to whom he can turn in confidence. "Dad is a bastard and I would never like to get his support. But John is such a great person and he gives me a lot of support. I can always count on him." Andrew knows that his mother is concerned about him and he feels support from her. But "I don't want to bother her with my problems."

Andrew's childhood was traumatic. His parents divorced when Andrew was three years old. Between the ages of six and nine he was sexually abused by his mother's new partner. Andrew's internal resources are limited: he has an almost nonexistent self-esteem, is dissatisfied with himself, turns aggressiveness inwards, and often feels sad and anxious. He seems to have some problems with writing and reading, difficulties in understanding certain words such as "self-blame," "neglect." Drugs and alcohol have become a "resource" to Andrew when he is confronted with problems.

The first year after the HIV diagnosis, Andrew withdrew socially and drank a lot. He feels that he was persuaded to be tested for HIV while being an in-patient at a psychiatric clinic. Today he strongly regrets that. Andrew feels that his life has "stopped, moved backwards" after the HIV diagnosis. Sometimes Andrew has suicidal ideation. On the other hand, he emphasizes that he will not fulfill other people's expectations of him to commit suicide, "I am not a shit who also commits suicide." Today he discloses his HIV status without any real discrimination, which brings him into difficult situations (e.g., being battered, stigmatized). Andrew reports intrusive HIV thoughts and feelings as well as strong AIDS ruminations. On the one hand, he is very afraid of becoming sick and on the other hand, he has a sense of mastery as to the HIV progression. With respect to coping styles, Andrew displays a combination of self-assertiveness and avoidance.

Chaos and emptiness characterize Andrew's internal world. There is a splitting between good and bad figures, between mistrust and idealization. Andrew, just like George, has a fragile self-image and a low self-esteem. He tries to compensate for this void by internalizing the idealized John, who represents strength and goodness. However, this compensation strategy make Andrew vulnerable and may manifest itself in anxiety attacks and psychosomatic symptoms. At the bottom line, Andrew experiences himself as Nobody, but the HIV infection makes him visible and provides him with a fragile identity, but still an identity. But there is a paradox here: the identity that makes him visible today may in the long run make him invisible again and destroy him. It is quite likely that the HIV infection reactivates the sexual abuse trauma. Both represent the threat of extinction. Since Andrew has such a low self-esteem, he internalizes (by means of John) a self-assertive attitude and in that way he gets at least a pseudo self-esteem. However, this attitude also functions as a manic defense against the powerful HIV. His avoidant coping style, just like drinking and other drugs, can be viewed as another desperate way to get away from HIV-related issues and mourning. Andrew's strong help-seeking attitude can be seen as a desperate hope that other persons will fill his internal emptiness but also in a magic way free him from the demon, the HIV infection.

Clinical Vignettes

The three renarratives offered below are based on the same gay men whose HIV disease scenario was presented in Chapter 8. Some details are excluded out of confidentiality, but that does not change the character of the renarratives.

Barry

When Barry starts in psychotherapy, he describes himself in negative terms and that he is "so terribly compliant with others—there is something weird with that." He also expresses guilt feelings related to sexuality but also has an avoidant attitude toward talking about sexual issues. The negative self-image in combination with his HIV seropositivity makes it extremely difficult—not to say impossible—for him to allow himself anything good in life. "Why should I—I'm going to die anyway, so why bother?" Another aspect he mentions, but does not want to address in any further details, is his fear of his fantasy world and of losing control. To Barry, losing control is equal to being or becoming "schizophrenic." During this first semester, another theme is Barry's disappointment in his mother's lack of mirroring him and his very strong negative feelings toward his father.

Barry attaches to the therapist, which induces guilt in him: "I'm really talking too much about myself—I feel sorry for you." The upcoming summer vacation evokes strong feelings of abandonment and grief, but also rage. "You better take with you my feelings when you take off for holiday." Barry's separation anxiety is also manifested in resistance: "I don't really know if I'm coming to the next session" (the last one before the vacation). He returns to the last session, but with strong resistance. Barry is reluctant to share with the therapist his feelings and thoughts during the session. "You've seen who I really am and now I'm closing myself, because I'm afraid that you won't be able to take any more from me." These words also reflect fear of attachment and its potential consequence in being abandoned. But by "closing" himself, Barry ends the semester with a sense of control.

Mirroring needs, attachment, and ambivalence color the second semester. Barry realizes that his compliant attitude toward others is a way to be mirrored—but a way he strongly questions during this semester. "You know, you have to pay a price—not to be true to yourself." He falls in love, which provides him with a sense of being confirmed and mirrored. Over the semester, Barry expresses more and more trust toward the therapist as she meets his mirroring needs. But it also becomes clear that the needy part of him triggers anxiety because of fear of rejection or abandonment. The needy part is manifested in the attachment to the therapist, "I wonder what it would be like having you as a mother," and Barry shares his fantasies and longing for symbiosis with the therapist. For example, he talks about his longing to stay in the therapist's office "forever" and that no other clients should "bother" their relationship. The other side of this symbiotic longing is Barry's fear to be "engulfed." When the therapist comes psychologically too close, he feels threatened and is afraid of not being good enough. A similar process, and in parallel to the psychotherapeutic one, takes place within the HIV scenario. Barry participates in a medical study but because of a decline in the CD4 he must resign from the study. He feels he has not been "good enough" and therefore he is "punished." His HIV concerns and feelings of being threatened by HIV are triggered as well as his fears to become rejected or abandoned by significant others due to his HIV infection.

Barry becomes aware of his ambivalence to attachment and can see that he in different ways tries to escape from his attachment to the therapist. One way is to test the therapist: "I'm like a teenager and in a rebellion toward my parents." Other ways are the internal distance approach (isolates the sessions), resistance, and psychologically shutting off the therapist. These different modes also help Barry become more independent. Toward the end of the second semester, Barry gets the insight that symbiosis is a lost paradise to which he cannot return. "It feels sad and it's painful that I have to give up that thought [of symbiosis], but I also feel relieved." When the second semester finishes Barry describes himself as "more independent, separate, and I have improved my skills in setting boundaries toward others." His trust and confidence in the therapeutic relationship is reflected in his words, "it goes without saying that I want to continue our work next semester."

During the third semester, Barry continues his struggle with independence: "I want to be separate but not secluded." He begins to ponder (in relation to the therapy) about his wish to try to "stand on my own feet," but he also expresses his ambivalence in terms of "do I really dare to leave the nest?" These thoughts also evoke "bad conscience." Another theme is his longing for intimacy. Barry talks about his internal struggle between on the one hand to be "self-sufficient" and on the other hand "being insatiable as to relationships." It is crucial to Barry to have a partner who also has HIV "because I'm so afraid to be rejected." Closely linked to his intimacy needs is his sexual depressiveness, which causes him psychological pain and despair.

Barry feels, as he says, increasingly attached to the therapist, which in turn triggers fantasies about symbiosis and fear of being engulfed. On the other hand, he experiences increasingly trust in the psychotherapeutic relationship and brings up childhood traumas. Barry also describes the therapist as "an internal support" to him when confronted with difficult or problematic situations.

The HIV scenario comes into an indirect play during this semester. Barry talks about his hope that he will still be around at his sixtieth birthday. "But I'm also aware that I might not live that long, but I still want to keep this hope." Thoughts about death enter the scene, which causes Barry a lot of pain and grief. "I don't want to die now."

In the final semester, Barry's own death becomes more salient in the sessions. He talks about arrangements for his own funeral and his wish to have friends at his bedside when he is dying. Barry reaches the existential insight (or existential death awareness) that the "definite separation" will come one day. As a result of a restored self with autonomy and clear boundaries, Barry decides to terminate psychotherapy. "I'm doing fine and I realize that I can handle my life much better now. I think I have achieved a lot and I have grown. I also know there are certain areas that I, at least for the time being, want to leave alone." He summarizes his psychological improvements in terms of "I'm more sensitive to my own needs, I feel secure and I'm much better in setting boundaries. I also feel that my self-confidence has increased." The psychotherapeutic relationship is summarized by Barry in the following way: "The continuity has been vital, just as being mirrored and respected by you have been decisive to my psychological growth."

Richard

At the beginning of the psychotherapeutic contact, Richard, who was then in the mild symptomatic phase, complains of not being seen and acknowledged by others. However, he is aware that his dissatisfaction goes many years back and he remembers that in his teens "I did anything to be seen."

He describes that there is a sense of only being approved of and liked when he performs well, "but these feelings have been with me for years." With respect to his gayness, he stresses that "I'm actually bisexual but that's something you can't speak about in the gay community." Richard perceives his mother as limitless, "well, she has a part in me being gay today." The father is described as "lovable but unpredictable because of his drinking and I was afraid of him when he was drunk."

Richard also perceives himself as having "relationship problems," and his "bad part and oppressive tendencies" frighten him. The most salient themes during this disease phase are his perceived disrupted mirroring needs, fear of attachment and of abandonment.

The disrupted mirroring needs are manifested in Richard's perception that "the hospital staff doesn't really see me. They don't respect me." There are also feelings of disappointment targeted at the staff, and in particular at physicians, expressed as "the medical care just deteriorates." Richard also conveys his dissatisfaction with his partner, who "does not support me enough."

Richard is aware of his fear of attachment and his tendencies to escape when the relationship gets "too close." "I have used my body and therefore I can't have intimacy." Eventually he realizes his clinging and demanding mode in intimate relationships and his easily evoked disappointed in other people. On the other hand, there is a longing for intimacy. "I want to have tenderness, closeness, and love." In the course of the psychotherapeutic work in the mild symptomatic phase, Richard is initially committed to a love relationship that eventually ends. Later, he gets involved in a new love relationship, in which Richard on the one hand feels good and "safe" and on the other hand controlled, isolated, and captured.

Richard describes the fear of attachment in terms of being "engulfed" and running the risk of being abandoned. However, it is also linked to the sense that "I've the idea that I'm not worthy to be loved and to have a good life." With respect to the attachment/abandonment theme, Richard talks about himself in terms of "I'm like a child looking into the house and then I feel so abandoned and alone."

HIV also triggers the fear of abandonment. Richard describes a medical examination situation, where he felt totally abandoned by the staff in that it did not provide him with any information regarding the examination. "It was just terrible." Richard also talks about his fear of becoming sick as it symbolizes to him "dependency" and the risk of being deserted. Just as afraid as he is to be ostracized and rejected because of HIV, this also has occurred to him, he sometimes experiences that people are too concerned about him "just because I'm HIV positive." This concern, however, evokes within Richard a sense of being reduced as a person, "I'm only a virus to them." When his partner breaks their relationship

Richard feels hurt, betrayed, and disappointed: "He couldn't cope with me being HIV positive."

Another theme that Richard reflects upon is his "difficulties to get sex and love together." There is a strong yearning within him to be "perceived as attractive on the sexual scene." He moralizes over his sexuality as expressed in words like, "it was sex without love and that's not the way it is supposed to be after you got your HIV diagnosis." He has some casual sexual encounters, which evoke guilt and shame: "I shouldn't behave like that when I'm HIV positive."

Richard attaches to the therapist, "I know, you are there for me," but he also underlines that "it's good there is a distance between the two of us." He wants her to be supportive of him in his official HIV-informant role, but sometimes the therapist is perceived as threatening. Richard also expresses ambivalence, but decides to continue the psychotherapeutic work when he starts on the AZT treatment.

Richard's mood oscillates during the mild symptomatic disease phase from depressiveness and pessimism to a good spirit. At the end of the disease phase, he says, "I feel happy, I'm at peace with myself and I'm more collected in myself."

The themes of fear of abandonment and perceived disrupted mirroring needs continue to be prominent during the severe symptomatic disease phase. But Richard's relationship to, in particular, his mother and control issues are also at the forefront. From time to time Richard fears being forgotten, feels alone and abandoned or neglected by friends and hospital staff as displayed in the following quotes: "I need to be seen," "The staff doesn't believe me in my feelings and experiences. They just ignore me," "The doctors don't inform me properly." During one of his hospitalizations, Richard remembers when he was in hospital as a kid and his mother did not visit him. This memory stirs up a lot of painful emotions and rage toward his mother. He also feels neglected by his siblings, who "don't give me the kind of support I need." The other side of the coin is that Richard is ambivalent toward social contact. It is manifested in that he on the one hand wants to withdraw because of his impaired health and on the other hand gets disappointed in friends who do not call him. "But I also realize that I have to pick up the phone, but I don't have the energy right now to do that." He also expresses disappointment in those who do not respect him in his social withdrawal. Not only fear of abandonment but also HIV triggers fear of extinction. Richard becomes aware of his tendencies to withdraw socially when people or HIV get too close to him.

Richard is quite occupied by his childhood and his role in the family. He was the "fixer," whose role was to understand others and "be a big ear to their needs," whereas Richard's feelings were of a second order. He describes feelings of being an outsider of the family in which the siblings' well-being took precedence over Richard's. He also talks about his fear of his father and his "boundless" mother. Richard's feelings and attitude toward his mother oscillate over the disease phases. At times, he expresses bitterness, disappointment, and rage toward and a sense of being deceived by his mother. However, Richard also reaches out to his mother and eventually he acknowledges that "this is the mother I have. Although we have a superficial communication there is a strong wish from both of us to maintain our relationship."

Control is another aspect that is of vital concern to Richard. He fears on the one hand to be controlled by others and on the other hand to lose control. It becomes important to Richard to be in control of his medication. When he is in control his psychological well-being increases. From time to time Richard experiences "aggressive outbursts" that frighten him, "you know, I'm just out of control then." He reflects over this and eventually he realizes that the outbursts are a projection of "the bad HIV" and behind it, there is despair, grief, and death anxiety. Richard also ponders a lot over his childlessness, which causes him pain and grief. He wishes he had children, "that would be a way to leave something of myself here on earth."

During the severe symptomatic disease phase, Richard gets involved in a new love relationship. As he becomes sicker, the relationship is confronted with multiple distresses of which the sexual sphere is one. Richard's sexual interest and desire declines, which is not a problem to him "but it becomes a problem because Roger wants to have sex." The therapist meets with the couple for few sessions that, according to the couple, strengthen their relationship.

Richard expresses his trust in the therapeutic relationship and his need "to be allowed to feel sad, distressed, miserable and as a child." He escapes from the contact during a period when he is doing fine physically. The therapeutic relationship intensifies when Richard gets sick and is hospitalized. He experiences severe anxiety, of which a large proportion relates to death anxiety and existential death awareness. These existential concerns trigger Richard's fear of being abandoned. Richard recovers and makes the comment "we made it, and we will make it in the future as well."

Richard becomes more aware that his physical state has an impact on his psychological well-being. Although he feels despair, helplessness, and grief, "I always try to find some positive things in my life. And these feelings don't feel as heavy as they used to." Toward the end of the severe symptomatic phase, Richard experiences a psychological equilibrium and his zest in life returns.

In the terminal phase, the psychotherapeutic contact is intense. Richard's mood swings between but also within the sessions; from being happy and in a good mood to the next moment of despair, grief, and helplessness. His need to be in control becomes salient. He is angry with the staff, and Richard directs his dissatisfaction upfront with the staff. There is ambivalence toward his love relationship, which he describes in terms of a child-adult relationship, Richard being the child. He also feels rejected by his partner. The therapist meets with the couple for a few sessions, and afterward they both express a sense of "having cleared the air."

As Richard's health further deteriorates, his death anxiety and existential death anxiety, but also his intimacy toward Roger, intensify. He talks about "the total separation," which fills him with grief, fear, and loss. Richard's death anxiety and existential death anxiety are reduced by means of his thoughts of returning to earth in another human being and through his intimacy to Roger.

Andy

Andy is in the asymptomatic disease phase when he starts psychotherapy. He describes a negative self-image in terms of feelings of guilt and shame related to his gayness, low self-esteem, and high performance anxiety; and he has no sexual encounters, which evokes grief. Andy summaries his self view as "I have no value and don't like myself." This negative self-image worsens in the second semester with feelings of emptiness, passivity, tendencies to isolate himself, and depressiveness. He also brings up his strong tendencies to comply with others and the gap between his intellectual and emotional spheres. At the end of the second semester, he becomes increasingly numb and depressed, "I'm like encapsulated in a cocoon," and he cries a lot. Andy expresses the wish of "having the bad removed" and his longing for a relationship. But for the time being "it [a relationship] is just out of the question," which makes him feel sad and full of despair. He is diagnosed with clinical depression and is put on antidepressants. He recovers and gets off the medication.

Andy employs an avoidant attitude toward HIV in that he does not want to talk about it and he has not disclosed his HIV serostatus to anyone. At the beginning of the therapeutic contact, Andy is somewhat skeptical because of earlier "bad experiences of therapists." The sessions are seen as parentheses to isolate what was going on in the sessions from one another, "but I have to take myself and my life seriously." During the second semester Andy attaches to the therapist and he perceives the sessions as "a breathing space." He also emphasizes that "I want to give myself a chance." At times, however, Andy perceives the therapist as dangerous and threatening and he is afraid of being abandoned by her. He talks about his worries that the therapist will "get tired" of him, and he asks, "Will you join me on my wandering? Imagine you abandon me in the dark forest."

Andy does not have a mild symptomatic phase as he was diagnosed in the third semester with AIDS. The most salient theme during the severe symptomatic disease phase is Andy's oscillation between a "bad" and a "good" self, which are also reflected in his mood oscillations. His "bad self" is very much characterized by a negative self-image, including shame and guilt related to sexuality and self-hatred toward his gayness. "I just can't respect myself." From Andy's perspective, he has no right to live and he experiences that no one "wants my goodness, I am just a bad guy." The "good self" is characterized by setting boundaries with others, feelings of being valued, liked, open to others, getting support and appreciation, and having the right to live. Andy experiences a period of "I'm surfing on the wave" including all the "good feelings," taking more responsibility in life, accepting himself, and experiences he has control over HIV and "I'll live another five years." During this period Andy discloses his HIV status to his family and starts to think about and to organize his funeral.

But as his health deteriorates further, his self becomes numb and empty, "there are no feelings inside me," with indifference and hopelessness. HIV is like a prison to Andy and his experience is that when he is "on permission from the prison," which happens "rarely," he gets access to his emotional world. Andy becomes increasingly depressed and is eventually diagnosed as clinically depressed and is put on antidepressants again. However, his sense is that: "I'm at the bottom of a hollow and I can't get out of it despite antidepressants and our relationship. But it feels good to have you with me at the bottom, that we share this." In the course of the severe symptomatic phase, Andy attaches strongly to the therapist, of which the above quote is one manifestation. The attachment is also reflected in his increased ability to express his feelings. Earlier in the disease phase, however, he is more ambivalent. He talks about the sessions as "they stir up too much," and he is afraid that the therapist won't be able to "hold" him. As time goes by Andy develops more trust in the therapeutic relationship and he says, "it really helps me to come to the sessions. Everything feels so much easier after seeing you and the sessions make me feel like there is a future and that's a good feeling." The therapeutic relationship intensifies as Andy gets sicker.

During this disease phase, Andy also brings up his intimacy difficulties. There is a longing for but also a fear of closeness and intimacy. Andy explains that he finds it very hard to show his grief and sadness within a relationship and that there are feelings of guilt and shame linked to intimacy. In the therapy, he acknowledges, with great pain, his longing to be liked and loved. He tells the therapist that he has not had any sexual encounters during the last four years and that he struggles with feelings of being "poorly sexually equipped." When Andy is diagnosed with AIDS, he becomes worried about being abandoned. He experiences that he is "not seen by the doctors." He socially withdraws for a while, but eventually he opens up to his social network.

Control issues is another theme as manifested in his strong conviction that "I have the right to decide over my life. And if I want to shorten it, it is up to me." Andy also realizes that his flight into work when feeling distressed is a way for him to control his emotions. However, he feels more and more alienated at work and struggles with whether to quit the job or not. Andy becomes aware that when he dares to let go of his emotions his psychological well-being improves.

At the beginning of the severe symptomatic phase, Andy talks about "a moment of death anxiety." As his health is further impaired, he talks more about death anxiety and death wishes but also about his longing for life: "I want to pull the emergency handle because I feel valued now and I want to live."

Entering the terminal phase there is still a longing for life. Andy wants to buy a dog, "which would make me feel good and I also would have to take responsibility." But there is also a longing for death "to put an end to all this." Andy becomes more introverted and declares his grief over having to say good-bye to his beloved friends and family. "I'm so sad that I'm not going to be old." He regains his "good" self, gives in, and resigns himself to both death and life.

REFERENCES

1. Abramowitz S, Cohen J. The psychodynamics of AIDS: A view from self psychology. In: Cadwell S, ed. *Therapists on the Frontline*. Washington D.C.: American Psychiatric Press 1994; 205–221.
2. Nilsson Schönnesson L. HIV infection: Trauma, psychic metabolism, and, psychological well-being. A study of 29 Swedish gay HIV-positive men. Unpublished report (in Swedish). Stockholm; 1993.
3. Alexander CJ, Nunno V. Narcissism and egocentricity in gay men. In: Alexander CJ, ed. *Gay and Lesbian Mental Health. A Sourcebook for Practitioners*. New York: Harrington Park Press; 1996.
4. Miller A. *Das Drama des begabten Kindes und die Suche nach dem wahren Selbst*. Frankfurt am Main: Suhrkamp Verlag; 1979.
5. Isay RA. *Being Homosexual. Gay Men and Their Development*. New York: Avon Books; 1989.
6. Friedman RC. *Male Homosexuality. A Contemporary Psychoanalytic Perspective*. New Haven, Connecticut: Yale University Press; 1988.
7. Bell A, Weinberg M. *Homosexualities. A Study of Diversity Among Men and Women*. New York: Simon and Schuster; 1978.
8. Winnicott DW. *The Maturational Processes and the Facilitating Environment*. New York: International Universities Press; 1965.
9. Cornett C. *Reclaiming the Authentic Self. Dynamic Psychotherapy with Gay Men*. Northvale, New Jersey: Jason Aronson; 1995.
10. Ericson EH. *Childhood and Society*. 2nd ed. New York: W.W. Norton; 1963.
11. Sullivan HS. *The Interpersonal Theory of Psychiatry*. New York: W.W. Norton; 1953.
12. Kertzner RM. Entering midlife: gay men, HIV, and the future. *Journal of the Gay and Lesbian Medical Association* 1997; 2(1):87–95.
13. Blechner M. The shaping of psychoanalytic theory and practice by cultural and personal biases about sexuality. In: Domenici T, Lesser R, eds. *Disorienting Sexuality*. New York: Rutledge; 1995; 265–288.
14. Isay RA. On the analytic therapy of homosexual men. *Psychoanalytic Studies of Children* 1985; 40:235–255.
15. Kohut H. *The Analysis of the Self*. New York: International Universities Press; 1971.
16. Charmaz K. The body, identity, and self: Adapting to impairment. *The Sociological Quarterly* 1995; 36(4):657–680.
17. Kidel M. quoted in Charmaz K. The body, identity, and self: Adapting to impairment. *The Sociological Quarterly* 1995; 36(4):657–680.
18. Nilsson Schönnesson L. Living with HIV. Dead end and/or turning point? In: Friedrich D, Heckman W, eds. *AIDS in Europe—The Behavioral Aspect*. Vol. 1, *General Aspects*. Berlin: Edition Sigma; 1995.
19. Silverstein C. The borderline personality disorder and gay people. In: Ross MM, ed. *Psychopathology and Psychotherapy in Homosexuality*. New York: Haworth Press; 1988; 185–212.

20. Nilsson Schönnesson L. *The Relationship Between Homosexuality and Psychological Functioning in a Perspective of Personality Types*. Stockholm: Almqvist & Wiksell International; 1983.
21. Dreifuss-Kattan E. *Cancer Stories. Creativity and Self-Repair*. Hillsdale, New Jersey: Analytic Press; 1990.
22. Langs R. *Death Anxiety and Clinical Practice*. London: Karnac Books; 1997.

10

Autonomy, Boundaries, Control, and Death

At the beginning of this book, we described its focus in terms of illuminating the drama of the HIV scenario and the psychological landscapes in which it is embedded among gay men with HIV. We believe that through the longitudinal, long-term study of the 38 gay men with HIV, we have been able to demonstrate that the psychosocial, sexual, and existential issues that emerged were more salient at different levels of the disease process. This would not have been possible by applying a cross-sectional approach, which is characteristic of most of the previous national and international studies. We also think that the study has illuminated many of the responses to, and impacts of, chronic and terminal illnesses discussed in Chapter 2. There is no doubt that the responses to and the adaptation processes of HIV disease scenario as well as the self scenario are a complex and multifaceted web. We also believe that with the exception of access to health care, an issue that sets the United States apart from all other civilized democracies, the psychological issues that arise in the Swedish sample can be shown to be almost identical to those that have been discussed in the literature from the United States.

While it is not possible to talk about one HIV drama in all temporal phases, we can say that the drama changes its gestalt in the course of the disease progress. These changes are not solely associated with physical but also with HIV-related psychological processes and the psychological landscapes. The latter refers to the individual's self, adaptation processes, and the existential context. We could thus argue that there are potentially as many HIV dramas as there are people living with HIV. Nevertheless, there appear to be consistent issues and themes that are shared by gay men with HIV, although their specific contents may vary from one person to another.

In Table 4, we summarize the psychological processes, including issues and themes, that were common for all four disease phases as well as those that were more salient at different levels of the disease process. However, because the individual and the pace of the disease progression through the stages will vary, they are a guide rather than a blueprint.

As the table shows, physical, psychological, and existential death-related themes and issues were of vital concern to the men during the whole course of the

Table 4. Summary of Psychological Processes over the Four HIV Disease Phases

	THE DISEASE PROCESS				
Psychological processes	All four disease phases	The asymptomatic phase	The mild symptomatic phase	The severe symptomatic phase	The terminal phase
Existential concerns	Thoughts of death; Existential death awareness; Death/indirect: limitations; Symbolic immortality; Loss of timelessness; Loss of life	Death/indirect: finitude, irreparable loss, boundaries; Meaning in life	Existential death anxiety; Death/indirect: boundaries; Longing for death; HIV concerns; Fear of psychological death	Existential death anxiety; Loss of life; Death/indirect: restrictions; Death symbols; Longing for death; After-death thoughts	Existential death anxiety; Loss of life; Death symbols; Existential guilt; Ambivalence; Mortal/immortal; Resignation
HIV threats	Insidious persecution Medication concerns; Loss of friends; Sexual concerns	Time; Self-disclosure	Bewilderment; Self-disclosure; Loss of friends	Fear	Confirmation; An outsider
Psychological issues	Aloneness; Control/uncertainty; HIV = limitations	HIV = finitude, irreparable loss, boundaries; Control issues; Decreased sexual interest/desire	Loss of body; HIV = persecutor, punishment, boundaries; Decreased sexual interest/desire	Loss of body, identity; HIV = prison, persecution, restrictions; Control issues	HIV = persecutor; Loss of body, identity; Aloneness

Mood	Anger; Helplessness; Hopelessness; Despair	Anger; Suicidal ideation; Worries	Anger; Worries	Suicidal ideation; Vulnerability; Imprisoned; Insulted; Helplessness; Hopelessness; Despair; Hope	Vulnerability; Disappointment; Violation; Helplessness; Hopelessness; Despair; Hope
Self issues	Shattered self	Vulnerable; Rejection; Internal intimacy conflicts; Mirroring needs	Vulnerable; Rejection; Internal intimacy conflicts; Mirroring needs; Dualism	Vulnerable	
Defenses	Avoidance; Magical thinking; Projection	Denial	Denial	"Rescuer" from death	"Rescuer" from death
Restored self	Increased sense of control, choice, vitality, and self-respect				

disease process. However, at the beginning of the disease process, death was talked about in an indirect way in terms of boundaries and finitude, whereas in the severe symptomatic and terminal phases death was related to both indirectly (e.g., death symbols) and directly (e.g., longing for death). Fear of psychological death was salient in particular during the mild symptomatic phase. The table also illustrates that the gay men in the terminal phase oscillated between the realization of being mortal and the sense of being immortal, and that they also employed an ambivalent attitude toward death.

Regardless of levels of disease process, the HIV infection was experienced by the men as an insidious persecutor, but its character changed over time. In the asymptomatic disease phase, the persecutor was related to time, whereas in the mild symptomatic phase, the persecutor caused bewilderment, and in the severe symptomatic phase, it caused fear. The insidious persecutory character of the HIV disease was confirmed in the terminal phase.

With respect to psychological issues, HIV represented limitations to the men regardless of where in the disease process they were. Control issues were more salient in the asymptomatic and the severe symptomatic disease phases and experiences of aloneness in the terminal phase. In the first two disease phases, the men experienced a decline in their sexual interest and desire.

Although feelings of helplessness, hopelessness, and despair were encountered over the whole disease process, they were in particular salient in the severe symptomatic and terminal phases, as was hope.

The shattered self, in terms of a vulnerable self, and in the asymptomatic phase as dualistic (i.e., dual self-perceptions) as well, was manifested in all phases except the terminal disease phase. The HIV infection appeared to trigger internal intimacy conflicts as well as mirroring needs in the asymptomatic and mild symptomatic phases.

The defense mechanism of denial was typical of the early phases of the disease, whereas the "death rescuer" defense was prominent in the severe symptomatic and the terminal phases. In addition, avoidance, projection, and magical thinking were recognized in all four disease phases.

Considering the protease inhibitor and other drug combination therapies, the reader might ask whether the synthesis presented here could be applied to the new situation. Since we lack data, there is not much we can say except point out that we need further research. However, based upon our current clinical experiences and anecdotes, we would suggest that the synthesis (at least parts of it) appears to be applicable even today. However, we have to pay attention to which "combination treatment group" of gay men we have in mind. We propose that those men who for example are newly diagnosed and asymptomatic may need to talk about their worries and uncertainties related to the medication (HIV threats). Another area of importance would be the existential one in terms of indirect manifestations of death such as limitations, restrictions, and boundaries. Although the new medication postpones HIV-related symptoms, it does not take away the infectiousness of the disease and thus sexual boundaries. In other words, regardless of new HIV treatment the individual faces sexual dilemmas (threat toward the sexual existence). Another potential existential concern would be the fear of psychological death and aloneness by means of stigmatization and discrimination (threat toward the social existence). Further, we believe that the new combination treatments can never take away the traumatic element of the HIV diagnosis and its attack on the individual's self. Therefore, we also have to be alert to the extent to which the gay man experiences a shattered self and his mirroring needs.

The situation of gay men who are long-term nonprogressors or long-term survivors is somewhat different. Many of them have struggled with the psychological processes described in Table 4. Protease inhibitors have become one more area of uncertainty to them and another condition that fosters a reevaluation of their view of life. Those men who have cycled through episodes of health and illness for years and now have regained health may feel psychological depletion. They may feel depleted of the ability to reintegrate into health, despite feeling physically sound and even able to restart work and psychosocial activities that they had abandoned.

FOUR CENTRAL PSYCHO-SOCIAL EXISTENTIAL ISSUES

Taking the above data together with the case vignettes, there are four central psycho-social existential issues that appear to emerge in most of the cases we have reported on here. These include mirroring issues, boundary issues, control issues, and existential and death issues. If we were to characterize the emergent issues in a mnemonic, we would call it "ABCDE"—Autonomy and self-worth, Boundaries, Control, Death, and Existential issues!

Death, Other Existential Issues, and Mirroring Issues

In common with people who are facing a potentially and foreseeable terminal illness, the gay men with HIV disease faced existential concerns and crises surrounding the meaning of life, responsibility, existential isolation, and death. The issue of death overshadowed the disease phases and the illness drama—its assured appearance in the final act leads to its implicit appearance throughout the whole play. It is strikingly similar to Beckett's[1] play *Waiting for Godot*, which centers around a character who is the focus of the dialogue while not actually appearing (and it is never certain whether or when he will appear). While we have noted indirect and direct death anxiety, we have also identified life anxiety, particularly in those men whose excellent response to protease inhibitors has lead to their having to consider continuing life as their problem rather than impending death.

However, HIV does not only physically threaten the individual's physical and psychological existence with death. The psychological existence is further threatened with death (i.e., to be or to become no one) by the fact that HIV seems to trigger internal intimacy conflicts. These conflicts also circle around psychological living or dying as they involve fear of being abandoned or engulfed. The mirroring needs and having them met can be viewed from an existential perspective as a way to counterbalance these psychological death anxieties. But the mirroring needs and their confirmation also have a psychodynamic function. They play a vital role in the restoration of the shattered self. HIV disease echoes other traumas, which together with HIV as such may destabilize and shatter the self. These traumas may be related to rejection because of one's sexual orientation by significant others and discrimination against both people with HIV and gay men, or rejection by a gay community focused upon youth and attractiveness for those who are aging or who do not meet with gay community definitions of attraction, including rejection by potential sexual partners because of an HIV-seropositive status. The primary need of therapy is to restore the shattered self to a sense of autonomy and self-worth.

Boundary and Control Issues

Boundary issues emerged in many guises. These ranged from the ultimate boundary of life and death to sexual boundaries symbolized by the condom or limits on sexual practices, social boundaries marked by discrimination, boundaries of disclosure marked by the shadow of the closet door, and boundaries of physical functioning imposed by the response of the body to disease. Such boundaries are perceived as obstacles in the individual's life as they are imposed upon him by HIV, that is, the external boundaries are manifestations of external control. On an existential level, external boundaries/control can be perceived as a representative of psychological death. Other boundaries, such as setting boundaries with disclosure in relationships, boundaries with the therapist and with lovers and families or friends, and boundaries of the self, are perceived as positive in that they impose order and structure to the individual's life (i.e., internal control). We also want to reiterate that not all the men had a lack of internal boundaries (or internal control) but they all struggled with setting or defining them better. However, these internal boundaries are also psychologically potential targets of HIV in that HIV attacks and destabilizes the self. As long as the internal boundaries are intact, they provide definition and a sense of certainty or control amid great uncertainty—indeed, they may be seen as a response to uncertainty. On the other hand, the ability to tolerate uncertainty is an essential part of "emotional maturity."[2] As the disease progresses, the individual increasingly perceives that he is losing internal control to external control (i.e., HIV), which is reflected in his feelings of helplessness, hopelessness, and powerlessness. Over all this is the wish of controlling the ultimate boundary, death. The therapeutic relationship is an example of the two sides of the boundary concept. On the one hand, the therapeutic relationship was perceived as certainty and continuity and supporting the client in keeping his internal boundaries. On the other hand, the therapy imposed control (death) by its therapeutic frame. In a symbolic way, the psychotherapeutic relationship represented life and death.

PSYCHOTHERAPEUTIC ISSUES

We have demonstrated that the psychological issues that face gay men with HIV disease are a process that moves with disease progression and are intimately bound up with existential concerns, in particular death. These concerns are to be expected and their salience is common, provided the psychotherapist or counselor has an intellectual and emotional awareness and openness toward them. Unfortunately, many psychotherapists and counselors are either poorly equipped to deal with these, or find them threatening. Professionals who deal with gay issues are often not conversant with death, dying, and other existential givens. Conversely, professionals who deal with people with chronic and terminal diseases are usually unfamiliar with gay lifestyle issues, stigmatization, and discrimination (at least as applied to gay subcultures). The close interweaving of both these issues, which cannot be separated, makes it important to examine their impact on gay men with HIV disease. It is thus an understatement that working with people living with HIV means that the psychotherapist and counselor become part of an emotionally powerful sphere. Schaffner[2] points out three major differences for the therapist/counselor working with people with HIV compared to more traditional psychotherapy or counseling: (1) The therapist/counselor has to focus on the myriad of external and internal realities of the individual's life; (2) The therapist/counselor is forced to work with special emotional stresses and discomforts that go with the grave unknowns and uncertainties of the individual's life. (S)he also has to learn about the profound damage inflicted on the HIV patients' life by stigma and how to relieve it; and (3) The therapist is personally challenged and required to reexamine his or her own values and conceptions of life, and we would add, other existential concerns as well as values of and attitudes toward sexuality and gayness. If these issues are not carefully worked through by the therapist/counselor, there is the risk that (s)he avoids (more or less unconsciously) the client's concerns, worries, and anxiety, in particular those related to dying and death. This leads us into the issue of countertransference.

Countertransference

Countertransference has been (like the concept of transference) much debated in the psychodynamic communities. One extreme stand believes that countertransference represents "eruptions of the psychotherapist's psychopathology"[3] (p. 159). The other extreme stand advocates that countertransference "encompasses all the feelings that the psychotherapist experiences in working with a patient"[3] (p. 159). In what follows, we only focus on countertransference issues that are specific to the HIV scenario. As it can be a personal challenge to work with people with HIV, it is important for the therapist/counselor to recognize and analyze the specific countertransference, which is an ongoing process.

Countertransference will impact therapists/counselors regardless of their sexual orientation, although in different ways. Gay-identified therapists risk over-identification with their clients or patients, which has been shown in work on HIV/AIDS-related health care worker burnout[4] to lead to problems in therapist coping and distress. It is not unusual for gay clients or patients to ask about the therapist's sexual orientation. This raises important issues, since the traditional approach of avoiding such discussion will also send a message. If the therapist is gay him- or herself and (s)he is uncomfortable about and unwilling to disclose him- or herself, it may be a reflection of the therapist's shame regarding her or his gayness. That in turn invites the client to feel ashamed of his gayness.[5]

Heterosexual therapists face equal but different countertransference issues. Perhaps the most important is their attitude toward gay men and people with HIV disease, which will become rapidly apparent to the client or patient. Any therapist who is uncomfortable with gayness should refer gay patients to another therapist who is more comfortable working with gays as soon as is ethically practical.

Where the therapist is HIV seronegative, then issues of survivor guilt may also arise, particularly if the therapist is gay and her/his case load is comprised largely of people with HIV disease. Where the therapist is him- or herself HIV seropositive, then the overwhelming nature of the client or patient's problems has obvious implications for countertransference. Another aspect is overprotection. The therapist has to guard his potential tendencies to overprotect the client in that it may jeopardize the psychotherapeutic work of restoring the client's sense of autonomy.

When the client/patient is dying it may evoke guilt feelings within the therapist/counselor that (s)he will survive the client. But the therapist/counselor may also have death wishes toward the client, so his (the client's) suffering and longing to die can end. These wishes in turn cause guilt in the therapist/counselor. One mode of protecting oneself from the guilt feelings is to identify with the dying client. On the other hand, the therapist feels ambivalence toward identifying with the client. The ambivalence can be manifested in different ways, such as the therapist missing sessions, or seeing the client on a more infrequent basis, or trying to calm the client with superficial comments, or starting to overprotect the client. It should be noted though that these mechanisms are of an unconscious character. As these feelings of ambivalence are inherent in working with terminally ill persons, they cannot be worked through.[6] As therapist/counselors, we have to become aware of and to understand feelings of ambivalence just as we must understand any death wishes toward the client. We need to have this awareness, otherwise we will not be able to holding the client and to provide the client with mirroring, twinship, and idealizing functions. The other side of the ambivalence is that if we cannot experience these feelings as well as feelings of love it becomes difficult to deal with the grief for the client we have come to care for so deeply (a caring that is consistent with an adequate empathic distance).

Supervision and Peer Support

As challenging and fulfilling as the work with people living with HIV is, it can also be draining, and the therapist's/counselor's self can be destabilized. It is not only the client's mirroring needs that have to be attended to. The therapist/counselor also needs to be confirmed in her/his mirroring needs to minimize the risk of burnout. As therapists/counselors we need to find ways to restore our selves. We all need to feel recognized, affirmed, and appreciated in our work. Working without supervision or peer support is dangerous both for the therapist and for their professional competence and development, as well as for their personal psychological well-being. The inevitable consequence of not being restored and affirmed is likely to be fatigue, depersonalization, and burnout.[4]

CLINICAL IMPLICATIONS

What are the implications of our findings for treatment and support of gay men with HIV disease? We will focus on three broader implications: first, the importance of the self in the HIV adaptation processes, second, application of these long-term and longitudinal data; and third, the role of the psychotherapist/counselor.

The Self and Its Role in the HIV Adaptation Processes

Based on our findings we want to underscore that a stabilized self is crucial to facilitate the approach and adaptation to the spectrum of HIV-related physical, social, and sexual threats, and psychological issues. We also believe that the vulnerable self may unconsciously play a vital role among some individuals, who are ambivalent toward taking HIV medication or incomplete in their adherence to the medical regimen. For example, if the person has a very low self-esteem or feels that he is unwanted or unloved, it might become difficult for him in the first place to accept, but also to retain, something "good" as the medication. In his own view, he is not worth it. If the individual accepts the medication out of his "mask of niceness" or his "impecable mask," the chances that he will not appropriately adhere to the HIV medication are quite high. The reason is that he accepts the treatment as a response to external control, that is, the individual behaves in a way he thinks it expected of him out of the wish not to be disliked. To be somewhat provocative, we would suggest the therapist/counselor question and initiate a dialogue related to medical adherence with those clients who just accept the medication without questioning it.

Having said that, we do not mean that every person with HIV should be in psychodynamically oriented insight psychotherapy. What we do propose is that by acknowledging and understanding the complexity of the individual's internal world and its impact on his external world, the psychotherapist/counselor will be able to adapt his therapeutic work to the client's distress and his resources. The overall objective of our therapeutic efforts, according to our view, is to guide and to support our clients in their fight for recapturing their autonomy, self-worth, self-esteem, and human dignity.

Application

The clinician who is dealing with large numbers of patients or clients may feel that we have had the luxury of seeing people over the long term. Dr. Schönnesson has seen the gay men on whom this book is based for periods ranging from one to seven years, with a mean of three years. However, we emphasize that much of this was intermittent, with these men attending as they felt it necessary or appropriate. Rather than this book making the point that long-term therapy is important (although it is so for some), we make the opposite point. If one can be clear about the issues that emerge and understand their interaction with disease phase, existential concerns, HIV-related threats and stressors better, then therapy or counseling can be both clarified and simplified. Paradoxically, the results of the long-term following of these men with HIV disease may make it less necessary for longer-term therapy. Traditional psychotherapy is also expensive, which few people with HIV can afford. Schaffner[2] argues that the treatment has to be modified to be more topic-focused "on the order of 'crisis intervention'."

Nor do we believe that for the counselor/therapist who is overwhelmed with a high case load, that individual therapy is the only avenue for treatment. It is our hope that the outlines of the issues in this book will contribute to constructing group therapy approaches from the presenting issues at various disease stages and related to classes of threats and stressors, or boundary imposition or setting. One purpose of this book has been to make the task of the psychotherapist/counselor easier in terms of clarifying the options available to them. Further, it may reduce the length of time that may be necessary to understand the presenting problems and the underlying themes with particular clients/patients. Again paradoxically, this long-term longitudinal work may make it possible for more streamlined approaches to provision of service.

The Role of the Psychotherapist/Counselor

No commentary on psychotherapy and counseling with gay men with HIV can bypass the difficulty posed by the impact of HIV infection on the brain and central nervous system, particularly in the later symptomatic stages of illness. In the more than 15 years we have both been working with gay men with HIV, we have noted that psychotherapists are often unlikely to consider that some psychological issues, such as mood disturbance or unusual reactions, may be the result of biological disease processes in the brain. We urge them to maintain a high index of suspicion for central nervous system involvement of the virus. By the same token, we have also noted that some medical personnel are equally unlikely to consider psychological factors in patients or clients. We urge them to consider the person as someone who is facing and grappling with major psychosocial stressors and to integrate this into their treatment of the whole person.

Lest this sound like a positivistic and therapist-centered approach to dealing with HIV disease in gay men, we want to emphasize that the locus of what is done is not the therapist or counselor, but the client. It has become increasingly obvious that HIV disease became, for many of the gay men, more of a psychological and existential work in progress than a minimally controllable trajectory of illness. It remains their work, not that of the therapist.

This book has been driven by the exploration of the themes, phases, threats, and distresses of the men we have worked with, and the locus of the knowledge and understanding we have gained remains with them. And we believe that the locus of "doing" should also remain with them. The role of the therapist/counselor, as we have indicated in the chapter on the self, is often most importantly to provide comfort and a supportive milieu in which the issues can be addressed. We have always taken the view that our expertise as therapists relates to seeing psychological improvement and increased quality of life in our clients or patients regardless of, and even independent of, their physical status. While the physician will inevitably have to face a sense of failure as patients get sicker and die, the psychotherapist can face a sense of success: that painful psychological issues have been successfully resolved, or at least rendered less painful. We need to emphasize that psychological insight and quality of life are unrelated to length of life. We can (paradoxically, if one is following a medical model) both be successful as therapists and have patients get physically sicker and die.

As psychotherapists/counselor we should strive to provide the person with HIV a holding environment or a safe space in which the individual can express and explore, among others, his fears, anxiety, fantasies, excitement, existential issues, dreams, grief, hope, bewilderment, anger, hopelessness, and joy. The most important gift we as psychotherapists/counselors can give the person with HIV is continuity, flexibility, and our accessibility. To quote Dreifuss-Kattan, we can:

> contain what has been put into me by the patient and so become the equivalent of a good mother, who provides a safe space, a framework, and a medium where the patient threatened by death can move freely between the illusion of union and the fact of separateness, as happens in the transitional phase of infancy.[6] (p. 212)

Finally, our intention was to provide the psychotherapist/counselor with the sort of insight that short time and high case loads are not always conducive to. Ultimately, however, its usefulness will be apparent not by the response of counselors and psychotherapists, but of the men who have been the focus of this work and who will be the final judges of its significance.

REFERENCES

1. Beckett S. *Waiting for Godot: A Tragicomedy in Two Acts*. London: Faber & Faber; 1965.
2. Schaffner BH. Modifying psychotherapeutic methods when treating the HIV-positive patient. In: Blechner MJ, ed. *Hope and Mortality. Psychodynamic Approaches to AIDS and HIV*. Hillsdale, N.J.: 1997; 63–80.
3. Cornett C. *Reclaiming the Authentic Self. Dynamic Psychotherapy with Gay Men*. Northvale, N.J.: Jason Aronson; 1995.
4. Bennett L, Miller D, Ross MW, eds. *Health Workers and AIDS: Research, Intervention and Current Issues in Burnout and Response*. London: Harwood Academic Publishers; 1995.
5. Isay RA. The homosexual analyst: Clinical considerations. In: Cornett C, ed. *Affirmative Dynamic Psychotherapy with Gay Men*. Northvale, N.J.: Jason Aronson; 1993; 177–198.
6. Dreifuss-Kattan E. *Cancer Stories. Creativity and Self-Repair*. Hillsdale, N.J.: Analytic Press; 1990.

Appendix

METHODOLOGY

The clinical data presented in this book stem from a quantitative and qualitative study of longitudinally psychotherapeutic notes of 38 gay men with HIV. It is important to note that the psychotherapeutic work was conducted without any intentions to use the case material for research purposes. The idea to transform the drama of HIV and its psychological landscapes into research was born in spring 1995 during Dr. Schönnesson's research visit as a Fulbright scholar at the HIV Center for Clinical and Behavioral Studies, Columbia University in New York.

The 38 gay men are part of a case load of 88 gay men living with HIV, all who have been in psychotherapy with Dr. Schönnesson. The psychotherapeutic work described here took place between 1986–1995 at the Ph center in Stockholm Sweden, a psychosocial center for gay and bisexual men with HIV-related problems run by the Stockholm city council. The purpose of the study was to longitudinally analyze and describe the meaning of living with HIV and the adaptation processes within a psychodynamic and existential perspective. The study was reviewed and approved by the Human Subjects Ethical Committee at Huddinge University Hospital, Stockholm.

The Sample

As thc purpose of the study was to examine meanings and psychological processes longitudinally, only those men who had had at least ten sessions were potential candidates (n = 65) for the study. These potential participants constituted three groups: Group 1: those men who in 1995 were in psychotherapy (14 men), Group 2: those men who had terminated psychotherapy (25 men), and Group 3: the deceased men (26 men). Because of ethical concerns, different approaches were used for each group in gathering informed consent. Group 1: The psychotherapist informed the men orally as well as provided them with a written informed consent form. Group 2: Those men who had terminated their therapeutic contact could not, out of ethical reasons, be contacted by the psychotherapist. Therefore, information about the study was distributed at various HIV medical centers in Stockholm, the Body Positive group, and through a printed advertisement in gay magazines. If the man approved of informed consent, he was asked to call the therapist or the secretaries at the Ph center. Group 3: The deceased group raised a delicate ethical concern. Considering the autonomy principle, it was decided to contact the partner and members of the original family, but only those who the psychotherapist had met (n = 14). She contacted them on the telephone explaining the study and a written informed consent form was also sent.

The potential sample comprised 53 men and the final sample consisted of 38 men (72%) of whom 14 were currently in psychotherapy, 10 had terminated their psychotherapeutic counseling, and 14 were deceased. There were no significant group differences as to age, year of HIV diagnosis, relationship status, reasons for contacting the center, earlier psychiatric consultation, or HIV disease phases. A staging classification was scored by Dr. Schönnesson on the basis on the individual's description of his health status to assign the client to a disease phase at his first visit with the psychotherapist. The asymptomatic phase (phase 1) refers to an "intact" immune system, no symptoms; the mild symptomatic phase (phase 2) a somewhat impaired immune system with mild symptoms; the severe symptomatic phase (phase 3) equals to a severely impaired immune system and severe symptoms, and finally the terminal phase (phase 4). The only significant difference was on the number of psychotherapeutic sessions. The men in the study sample had had more sessions compared to those who did not respond.

Two-thirds of the men started their psychotherapeutic work within a year of their first contact with the center. The others had had contact with a colleague at the center (at least one year) before they came to the psychotherapist. The mean year when the first contact was established with Dr. Schönnesson was in 1990 (range 1987–1995). All the men defined themselves as gay. The median age was 31 years (age range 18–58) and over one-half of them were single. The year of first finding out about their HIV seropositivity ranged from 1982–1993 with both a mean and median year of 1986. Almost one-half of the men (18 men) were in the asymptomatic phase and the mild symptomatic phase (17 men) respectively, two were in the severe symptomatic, and one in the terminal phase when the psychotherapeutic work started. These numbers of course changed over time and at the end of the study, the maximum cumulative number ever in a disease phase was 18 men in phase 1, 29 men in phase 2, 16 men in phase 3, and 13 men in phase 4.

The most frequent self-reported reasons for seeking professional help at the center were in descending order: HIV-related concerns, anxiety/depression, social concerns, intimacy concerns, substance use, and sexual concerns. None of the men asked for individual psychodynamic insight psychotherapy but rather expressed their needs to "talk to someone."

The years of being in psychotherapy ranged from one to seven years with a mean of three years. Considering this length of time, it is important to note that there were differences in intensity of sessions between the men as well as within the same man over the years. The total number of psychotherapeutic sessions varied between 11 to 177 with a median of 57 sessions.

Quantitative and Qualitative Analyses

The psychotherapeutic notes were analyzed both qualitatively and quantitatively. The first step in the analytic process was creating a codebook to be used as a tool in rating the clinical notes. These had always been made right after the session and consisted of the content of the session, which was decided by the client. The notes also consisted of those clarifications or interpretations that were shared with the client during the session. No clarification or interpretation that was not shared with and validated by the client during the session was recorded. Interventions were also noted in the records.

Dr. Schönnesson initially examined six sets of notes at random to determine the most common themes and domains. The codebook encompassed the following themes: HIV-related areas, non-HIV specific areas, homosexuality, relationships (including partner), existential aspects, moods, depression, anxiety, and suicide. Each theme and its domain had a number to be used in the coding of the case material. For example, 1121 referred to "disclosure of HIV to mother," 1141 to "on AZT, Videx, Hivid," and 233 referred to "hopelessness."

In the second step, Dr. Schönnesson and psychotherapist and sexologist Dr. Kerstin Fugl-Meyer, Department of Sexology, University Hospital of Uppsala, independently read each session of each client's chart and, using the codebook, coded its content. Additional themes and domains were added if necessary. A very high degree of inter-rater reliability was noted. Eva Edvardson, secretary at Ph center, then entered the coded session sheets into an SPSS file by semester (based on half-year semesters). Dr. Curtis Dolezal, HIV Center for Clinical and Behavioral Studies, Columbia University, New York, organized the data by disease phase and conducted quantitative analyses, including frequency analyses, paired T-tests analysis of themes by disease phase, and Pearson correlation coefficients.

The third step employed the qualitative data analysis of an in-depth case study for each client. Qualitative data analysis consists, according to Spradley,[1] of a search for the parts of a concept, the relationship between those parts, and the relationship of the parts to the whole. We followed this model using theme analysis. A theme is a pattern of thought that connects domains, and something that people within the target area will accept as valid. A domain is considered to be a symbolic category that contains related words. In many cases, the themes of a content area such as self or death may not be explicitly expressed and hence must be uncovered by the actions and descriptive language and rules of the target group. As data collection continues, the researchers continue to modify and add new domains based on comparison with previous data. Theme analysis occurred after data collection was completed. After identified domains, possible unidentified domains, descriptive examples, and other data were noted, the existing domains were compared and contrasted in order to find the themes and organizing domains.

The case study, which was organized by both semesters and disease phases, was based on the themes, domains, and affects described above together with data in the chart notes related to the self and the therapist-client relationship as well as quotes from the client. A phenomenological analysis of sentences by line was then carried out. Again, this coding was undertaken by Dr. Schönnesson and Dr. Kerstin Fugl-Meyer independently. Sentences were classified by labeling phenomena with key words without any interpretations by the raters. These key words ("at face value") were then categorized into concepts (e.g., self-image, conflicts, HIV representation) that seemed to pertain to the same phenomena. Again, a very high inter-rater reliability was obtained. In the qualitative analyses, the client's voice was extracted for direct use as quotes in the relevant section of the discussion.

The names that appear in the text are of course not actual names. We selected these names by taking a page of the *New York Times* and extracting first names by reading up from the bottom right-hand corner. These names were then applied sequentially to quotes.

REFERENCE

1. Spradley JP. *The Ethnographic Interview*. Fort Worth: Holt, Rinehart & Winston; 1979.

Index

MIX
Papier aus verantwortungsvollen Quellen
Paper from responsible sources
FSC® C105338

If you have any concerns about our products,
you can contact us on
ProductSafety@springernature.com

In case Publisher is established outside the EU,
the EU authorized representative is:
Springer Nature Customer Service Center GmbH
Europaplatz 3, 69115 Heidelberg, Germany

Printed by Libri Plureos GmbH
in Hamburg, Germany